THE COMPLETE
RENAL DIET
COOKBOOK
COLLECTION

with

The Best Renal Diet Recipes From The Complete Renal Diet Cookbook & Renal Slow Cooker Cookbook

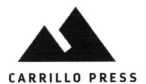

CARRILLO PRESS

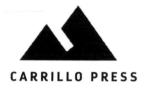

CARRILLO PRESS

CONTENTS

MEAT | 70

VEGETARIAN & VEGAN | 91

SEAFOOD | 110

POULTRY | 187

VEGETARIAN AND VEGAN | 198

INTRODUCTION

Welcome to The Renal Cookbook Collection!

This is the ultimate collection of over 170 recipes from both books in the series of Renal Diet Cookbooks from Carrillo Press; The Complete Renal Cookbook and The Renal Slow Cooker Cookbook.

We have combined all of the recipes in these two books to provide you with plenty of inspiration and meals to keep you going for weeks and months. Going through kidney disease can be hard enough at the best of times, without having to stress about the foods you're eating and the meals to cook. These recipes have been created with renal-friendly ingredients to help bring enjoyment to cooking as well as eating again. There are plenty of breakfasts, entrées, desserts and drinks to choose from, and if your lifestyle is a little hectic try any one of the 50 slow cooker recipes included. Each recipe is listed with important nutritional information, helping you to plan out your meals according to your specific needs.

As well as the recipes, we've included an overview of kidney disease and its different stages and the possible causes and potential symptoms you may be experiencing. The shopping and food lists aim to help you stock up your kitchen with essential items. Furthermore, we hope that the eating out and traveling advice will provide you with the confidence you need to continue socialising and doing the things you love again, whilst experiencing the earlier stages of the disease.

Whether you or someone you know has been diagnosed, you think you may be suffering from the symptoms but are not sure, or if you have a family history of chronic kidney disease and want to find out more about it, the good news is that with the right diet, medication and lifestyle, it is possible to delay and even prevent the need for dialysis and kidney transplants. It is always absolutely vital that you use this information alongside professional guidance; make sure you see your doctor if you have, or suspect you may have, kidney disease. It's also essential you continue to see your doctor, nutritionist or nephrologist regularly after your diagnosis and consult them before you make any dietary or lifestyle changes.

We wish you all the best in the kitchen and in health!
The Carrillo Press Team

1

THE TRUTH ABOUT KIDNEY DISEASE

Our kidneys perform vital functions in our body to help keep us healthy; they help to maintain mineral levels such as potassium, sodium and phosphorous as well as regulate water levels. Not only this but they remove waste and extra fluids from our body after digestion, exposure to certain medications and chemicals - and even after muscle activity. The enzyme renin, produced by the kidneys, helps to regulate blood pressure and create erythropoietin, thus triggering red blood cell production. Last but not least, our kidneys generate an active vitamin D that we need for healthy bones.

If left untreated, kidney disease could lead to kidney failure. Treatment for kidney failure is usually dialysis or a kidney transplant. However, kidney disease can be slowed down and treated with the right balance of medication, nutrition, and advice from your professional consultant.

CAUSES OF KIDNEY DISEASE

High blood pressure and diabetes (both type 1 and type 2) are the top two cause of kidney disease. However, if you do have diabetes, this can be controlled by monitoring blood sugar levels in order to help to prevent kidney disease as well as coronary heart disease and strokes.

Other causes include:

- Immune system diseases such as lupus, hepatitis B and C, and HIV,
- Frequent urinary tract infections affecting your kidneys (pyelonephritis) could cause scarring, which can lead to kidney damage,
- Inflammation of the glomeruli (the tiny filters inside the kidneys) can occur after strep infections,
- An inherited kidney disease called polycystic kidney disease causes fluid filled cysts to form in the kidneys,
- NSAIDS drugs such as naproxen and ibuprofen used for a prolonged period of time can permanently damage the kidneys,

- Taking illegal drugs such as heroin,
- Long-term exposure to certain chemicals can cause the breakdown of kidney functions.

If you experience kidney disease for longer than three months and it goes untreated then you will develop chronic kidney disease. Often, the symptoms of kidney disease can go unnoticed and therefore this can be dangerous as some patients develop chronic kidney disease without even being aware of having the earlier stages of kidney disease.

ACUTE RENAL FAILURE

If you experience a sudden, total loss of kidney function, this is known as acute renal failure. There are three top causes of renal failure:
1. A lack of blood reaching the kidneys,
2. Urine not being expelled from the kidneys and,
3. Direct damage to the kidneys.

There are several factors that can cause these three things to happen including:

- Traumatic injuries causing severe blood loss,
- Sepsis (an infection that can cause the body to go into shock),
- Severe dehydration (particularly in athletes because of the sudden breakdown of muscles and the release of large amounts of a protein called myoglobin that causes harm to the kidneys),
- An enlarged prostate,
- Drug/toxins,
- Eclampsia/pre-eclampsia/HELLP Syndrome in pregnant women.

SYMPTOMS OF KIDNEY DISEASE

There are many different symptoms that you may experience with kidney disease and these include:

- Fatigue,
- Loss of appetite,
- Difficulty concentrating,
- Sleep problems,
- Needing to urinate more frequently,
- Blood in urine,
- Foamy urine,
- Muscle cramps or twitches,
- Swelling in the ankles or feet (edema),
- Dry or itchy skin,
- Puffiness around your eyes.

Experiencing one or more of these symptoms may be an indication that you have kidney disease and you should consult a professional if you do experience any of the above. As these symptoms may also be a result of another illness or disease, kidney disease can often go unnoticed. It is even more important you ask your doctor about kidney disease if you do suffer from diabetes or high blood pressure, if you have a family history of kidney disease, or are over 60 years old.

Symptoms of acute renal failure include:

- Shortness of breath due to fluid build up,
- Reduced amount of urine,
- Ongoing nausea,
- Weakness,
- A pain or intense pressure on your chest.

Remember the only way of knowing you have kidney disease at any stage is through consulting a professional who will conduct a urinalysis, measure urine volume, take blood samples or use ultrasound to diagnose you. It is vital once you have been diagnosed that you follow professional advice in order to prevent renal failure. This will usually involve a combination of medications, a healthy lifestyle and a reduction of over the counter medications such as aspirin as well as removal of toxins in the home e.g. tobacco and cleaning products.

FIVE STAGES OF KIDNEY DISEASE

The different stages of kidney disease are determined by the glomerular filtration rate (GFR). This is the process where the kidneys filter the blood that removes fluids and wastes. The GFR calculation determines how well the blood is being filtered.

The GFR is calculated using a formula that includes your age, race, gender, and serum creatinine levels. The lower the number, the further along your kidney disease will be. For example, a GFR under 60 might indicate kidney disease. As always, this would have to be monitored and diagnosed by a professional.

Stage 1 kidney disease: GFR = approximately 90+

At this stage, you may not have any symptoms and so this is why it is often unnoticed. If your doctor does determine you have stage 1 chronic kidney disease it will usually be due to diabetes or high blood pressure. If there is a family history of polycystic kidney disease, you have a greater chance of experiencing chronic kidney disease and so it is wise to go for check ups to ensure you do not have kidney disease, especially if you suffer from any of the symptoms in the previous section.

Stage 2 kidney disease: GFR = 60-89

Symptoms in stage 2 might include higher levels of urea or creatinine in your blood; there may be protein or blood in your urine.
Treatments: if diagnosed at this stage your doctor or nephrologist will recommend suitable treatment including medication and a healthy diet and lifestyle. The goal is to keep the kidneys functioning healthily on their own for as long as possible and to potentially avoid having to go through dialysis or a kidney transplant by preventing the later stages of kidney disease.

Stage 3 kidney disease: 3a GFR = 45-59
3b GFR = 30-44
This stage is classed as moderate kidney damage. Waste products will start to collect in the blood, which can cause uremia as the kidney function declines. This

makes it more likely for you to develop kidney disease complications such as bone disease, anemia, red blood cell shortage, or high blood pressure.

At this stage you may start to experience kidney pain in your lower back as well as sleep problems due to cramps in your legs. Fatigue is more common at this stage, along with swelling of extremities or edema, shortness of breath, and fluid retention. You might notice changes in your urine such as a foamy consistency or changes in color to red, tea-colored, dark orange, or brown. Urination frequency may change.

Treatments: As Stage 3 kidney disease progresses it is recommended that you see a nephrologist who will perform a number of tests on your kidneys; you may also be sent to a dietician to help with your nutrition and meal plans.

If you have high blood pressure, your doctor will likely prescribe medicine. ACE inhibitors and angiotensin receptor blockers have shown the potential to slow down kidney disease progression in people who don't suffer from high blood pressure. You should ask your doctor about your medications and take them only as prescribed.

You need to make sure you are taking your medicines, eating healthily, not smoking and exercising regularly to help prolong your kidneys. Talk with your doctor about an exercise plan. Your doctor can also help you stop smoking.

Kidney disease can't be cured but by following doctor's orders you can slow down its progress.

Stage 4 kidney disease: GFR = 15-30

At this stage, waste collects in the blood causing uremia as kidney function decreases. Complications such as high blood pressure, cardiovascular disease, heart disease, anemia, and bone disease are likely to develop.

Treatments:

Appointments with your nephrologist are essential at least once every three months. They will conduct tests for creatinine, calcium, phosphorus, and hemoglobin levels to ascertain how well the kidneys are functioning. They will also monitor your blood pressure and diabetes if applicable. The ultimate goal is to keep your kidneys functioning for as long as possible, but it is also possible that they may start to prepare your body for dialysis. There are two main forms of dialysis:

1. Hemodialysis dialysis can be conducted either at a center or in your home by a care partner. The dialysis machine will remove some of your blood through an artificial kidney or dialyzer to clean out the toxins that your kidneys can't remove any more. The cleaned blood is then returned to your body.

2. Peritoneal dialysis is needle free and you don't need anyone to assist you.

The last option would be to have a kidney transplant.

Stage 5 kidney disease: GFR = 15 or below

This is end stage kidney disease. The kidneys will have lost all function and will not be able to work effectively. You will need a kidney transplant or dialysis to survive.

With stage 5 kidney disease you might experience increased skin pigmentation, tingling of your hands or feet, muscle cramps, swelling around your eyes or ankles, little or no urine flow, unexplained itching, problems concentrating, and fatigue.

You might start feeling better once you begin dialysis. By removing the toxins from the blood, and taking prescribed medications, you may still be able to emjoy a good quality of life.
If a kidney transplant is recommended or desired, your nephrologist will explain the process to you and get your name on a waiting list for a donated kidney or help you to find a living donor.

2

RENAL DIET AND NUTRITION

How can diet affect symptoms of kidney disease?

Changing your diet and lifestyle can go a long way in helping you control your kidney disease and preventing the later stages. This chapter will explore the different food and nutrient groups to consider when experiencing kidney disease.

Carbohydrates should make up the majority of your diet, as they're the primary source of energy for your body.
There are two types of carbohydrates: complex and simple. An example of a simple carbohydrate is fruit. Fruit is packed with fiber, vitamins and energy that your body needs. Examples of complex carbohydrates are grains, breads, and vegetables. All these carbohydrates provide minerals and vitamins as well as energy and fiber. Carbohydrates also play a vital role in balancing blood-sugar levels.

Protein repairs tissue and builds muscle. Your body also uses protein to build antibodies. These are your body's defense against disease. Animal foods are the primary sources of protein such as milk, beef, eggs, chicken and pork. Protein can also be found in some plants, legumes, nuts, and soybean products. Vegetables also contain small amounts of protein. Protein is essential for good health, however in later stages of chronic kidney disease your renal dietitian may have you cut back on protein intake. This is in order to help reduce stress on the kidneys from protein waste building up in the blood.

Fats transport vitamins K, E, D, and A to your cells. They produce the hormones testosterone and estrogen. Some fats have fatty acids that are good for your skin. These fatty acids also make up linings of cells in the body and help with the transmission of nerves. However, too much fat or the wrong kind of fat in your diet can cause weight gain, leading to heart disease and many other problems with your health.

There are two types of fats: unsaturated and saturated. Meat and dairy products are saturated fats. Too much of these fats can elevate your cholesterol, especially the LDL or low-density lipoprotein. This cholesterol is what causes heart disease and clogged arteries. The food and drug administration recommend reducing your saturated fat intake. Nuts, fish, and certain oils are good sources of unsaturated fats and all help to reduce cholesterol. Trans fats will raise cholesterol levels and your LDL just like saturated fats. The FDA suggests you choose food that is low in trans fats and saturated fats. Processed foods usually contain trans fats.

Sodium, potassium, and phosphorus are the three main minerals balanced by the kidneys. As chronic kidney disease gets worse, some foods will need to be avoided. Your kidneys will no longer be able to get rid of the excess from these minerals that you get from food. Blood tests will be conducted to monitor the levels of these minerals.

Sodium

In the early stages of kidney disease, a low sodium diet may be all you need if you have high blood pressure. Your kidneys cannot get rid of excess fluid and sodium from your body whilst experiencing kidney disease.

Just one teaspoon of salt, this includes sea and kosher salt, has 2,300 mg of sodium which is more than your daily allowance. To help identify salt in foods look for words on the label such as baking powder, sodium or brine in the ingredients list.

Generally, children and adults should eat less than 2,300 mg of sodium a day. If you are over 51, have diabetes, are African American, have chronic kidney disease or hypertension, you need to lower your sodium intake to 1,500 mg a day.

Potassium

Kidneys usually get rid of excess potassium in your urine to maintain normal levels in your blood. When experiencing kidney disease they can no longer do this effectively.
Hyperkalemia or high potassium occurs in people in advance stages of kidney disease. Symptoms of high potassium are a slow pulse, numbness, weakness, and nausea.

Phosphorus

Since your kidneys can no longer remove phosphorus from your blood and urine, hyperphosphatemia or high phosphorus may become a problem during stage 4 or 5 kidney disease.

3
RENAL DIET AND LIFESTYLE GUIDANCE

1. Follow Your Dietician's Advice!
During kidney disease this is extremely important. They can advise you on sodium content of favorite foods and give you recommendations on how to reduce your sodium intake. Your diet will be tailored to you, taking into account the stage of kidney disease and any other illnesses or diseases you suffer from.

2. Keep a Food Diary
You should track what you're eating and drinking in order to stay within the guidelines and recommendations given to you. Apps such as myfitnesspal make this extremely easy and even track many of the minerals and levels of sodium etc. in each meal.

3. Read Food Labels
•   Some foods have hidden sodium even if they don't taste salty. You will need to cut back on the amount of canned, frozen, and processed foods you eat. Check your beverages for added sodium.
•   Check food labels to avoid Potassium chloride, Tetrasodium phosphate, Sodium phosphate, Trisodium phosphate, Tricalcium phosphate, Phosphoric acid, Polyphosphate, Hexametaphosphate, Pyrophosphate, Monocalcium phosphate, Dicalcium phosphate, Aluminum phosphate, Sodium tripolyphosphate, Sodium polyphosphate.

4. Flavor foods with fresh herbs and spices:
• These add flavor and variety to your meals and are not packed with sodium; spices also have many health benefits! Try these instead of salt and bottled salad dressings.
• Stay away from salt substitutes and seasonings that contain potassium.
• Use citrus fruits and vinegars for dressings and to add flavor.

5. Keep up your appointments with your Doctor or Nephrologist:
- Let your doctor know if you notice any swelling or changes in your weight.
- Meet with a dietitian to set up a plan based on your individual needs as well as your blood tests.

6. Be mindful of what you're eating:
- Be careful when eating in restaurants -ask for dressings and condiments on the side and watch out for soups and cured meats.
- Watch out for convenience foods that are high in sodium.
- Prepare your own meals and freeze them for later use.
- Drain liquids from canned vegetables and fruits; this will help control potassium levels.
- Measure portion sizes: moderating your portion sizes is essential. Use smaller cups, bowls, or plates to avoid giving yourself oversized portions.
- Visual Guides:
- The size of your fist is equal to 1 cup.
- The palm of your hand is equal to 3 ounces.
- The tip of your thumb is equivalent to 1 teaspoon. A poker chip is equal to 1 tablespoon.

7. Monitor drink and fluid intake:
You have probably been told you need to drink up to eight glasses of water a day. This is true for a healthy body but for people with chronic kidney disease in the later stages these fluids can build up and cause problems. The restriction of fluids will differ from person to person.
Things to take into consideration are: swelling, urine output, and weight gain. Your weight will be recorded before dialysis begins and once it's over. This is done to determine how much fluid to remove from your body. If you are undergoing hemodialysis, this will be done approximately three times a week. If you are undergoing peritoneal dialysis, your weight is recorded every day. If there is a significant weight gain you may be drinking too many fluids.

8. Substitution Tips:
- Use plain white flour instead of whole-wheat/whole-grain
- Use all-purpose flour instead of self-raising,
- Use Stevia instead of sugar,
- Use egg whites rather than whole eggs,
- Use almond, rice or soy milk instead of cows milk.

FOODS TO AVOID:

- Cured meats

- Bacon and ham

- Canned fish

- Cold cuts

- Frozen dinners

- Salted nuts

- Canned beans with salt added

- Canned entrées

- Bananas

- Raisins

- Oranges

- Cantaloupe

- Pumpkin

- Potatoes

- Dried beans

- Tomatoes

- Yogurt

- Ice Cream

- Milk

- Nuts and seeds

- Salt substitutes

- Molasses

- Chocolate

- Bottled coffee drinks

- Non dairy creamers

- Cereal bars

- Enhanced chicken and meat

- Sodas

- Iced teas

- Flavored waters

- Sardines

- Offal

- Processed meats

- Corn

- Dried beans

- Nuts and nut butters

- Avocado

- Pizza

- Biscuits, pancakes, waffles

- Corn tortillas

- Whole grain crackers, breads, cereals

- Brown or wild rice

- Bran

- Chocolate

- Beer, chocolate drinks, cola, milk-based coffee

- Ice cream

- Yogurt

- Cheese

- Milk

- Salted Butter

- Coconut

- Powdered coffee creamer

- Solid shortening

- High potassium fruits should be avoided. A serving of the following listed fruits has more than 250 mg of potassium:

- 5 dried prunes or ½ cup prune juice

- 1 small banana

- 1/8 of a honeydew melon

- ¼ cup dates

- ½ cup orange juice or 1 small orange

- 1 small nectarine no bigger than 2 inches across

- 5 dried apricots or 1 cup canned or fresh apricots

These vegetables have more than 250 mg of potassium in each 1.2 cup serving:

- Fresh beets

- Winter squash

- Tomatoes, juice, or ¼ cup sauce

- Sweet potatoes

- Spinach

- Potatoes

- Okra and Brussel sprouts

- ¼ avocado or 1 whole artichoke

FOODS TO ENJOY:

Red bell peppers have low potassium but lots of flavor. They are also a good way to get folic acid, fiber, vitamin C, A, and B6. Red bell peppers also contain lycopene - an antioxidant that helps protect against cancer. A ½ cup serving contains 10 mg of phosphorus, 88 mg of potassium and 1 mg of sodium.

Cabbage contains phytochemicals - a chemical compound found in fruits and vegetables that helps break up free radicals. Phytochemicals are known to protect against cancer and help keep your heart healthy. Cabbage is high in vitamin C, K, B6, folic acid and fiber. A ½ cup serving contains just 9 mg of phosphorus, 60 mg potassium, and 6 mg sodium.

Cauliflower contains indoles, glucosinolates, and thiocyanates. These help the liver get rid of toxins that could damage cell membrane and DNA. A ½ cup serving of boiled cauliflower has 20 mg phosphorus, 88 mg potassium, 9 mg sodium.

Garlic helps reduce inflammation, keeps plaque from building on your teeth, and lowers cholesterol. Just one clove of garlic has 4 mg of phosphorus, 12 mg of potassium and 1 mg of sodium.

Onion contains quercetin an antioxidant that protects against cancers and helps heart disease. Onions contain chromium - a mineral that helps with protein, carbohydrate and fat metabolism. A ½ cup serving has 3 mg phosphorus, 116 mg potassium, and 3 mg sodium.

Apples prevent constipation, reduce cholesterol, reduce the risk of cancer, and protects against heart disease. Apples have anti-inflammatory compounds and are high in fiber. Just 1 medium apple with skin on has no sodium, 158 mg of potassium and 10 mg of phosphorus.

Cranberries can keep you from getting a bladder infection because they prevent bacteria from sticking to the bladder wall. Cranberries can also help the stomach from creating the bacteria that causes ulcers thus promoting good GI health. Cranberries can also protect against heart disease and cancer. A ½ cup cranberry juice cocktail has 3 mg phosphorus, 22 mg potassium, 3 mg sodium. A ¼ cup of cranberry sauce has 6 mg phosphorus, 17 mg potassium, and 35 mg sodium. A ½ cup of dried cranberries has 5 mg phosphorus, 24 mg potassium, and 2 mg sodium.

Blueberries help reduce inflammation. Blueberries contain manganese, fiber, and vitamin C. They also help protect the brain from the effects of aging. A ½ cup of fresh blueberries has 7 mg phosphorus, 65 mg potassium, and 4 mg sodium.

Raspberries contain phytonutrient ellagic acid which helps reduce free radical cell damage. They are high in vitamin C, manganese, folate, and fiber. A ½ cup of raspberries has 7 mg phosphorus, 93 mg potassium, 0 mg sodium.

Strawberries are a good source of manganese, vitamin C, and fiber. They provide anti-inflammatory and anti-cancer compounds and help to protect the heart. A ½ cup or 13 mg phosphorus, 120 mg potassium, 1 mg sodium.

Cherries when eaten daily can help reduce inflammation.. A ½ cup serving of fresh cherries has 15 mg phosphorus, 160 mg potassium, 0 mg sodium.

Red grapes protect against heart disease by reducing blood clots. They also help protect against inflammation and cancer. A ½ cup red grapes has 4 mg phosphorus, 88 mg potassium, 1 mg sodium.

Egg whites contain the highest quality protein and essential amino acids. 2 egg whites contain 10 mg phosphorus, 108 mg potassium, 110 mg sodium, and 7 grams protein.

Fish is a source of protein and anti-inflammatory fats known as omega-3s. Omega-3s help fight heart disease and cancer. It is recommended that you eat fish two times a week. Try mackerel, salmon, rainbow trout, albacore tune, and herring. A 3 ounce serving of wild salmon has 274 mg phosphorus, 368 mg potassium, and 50 mg sodium.

Olive oil helps fight against oxidation and inflammation. Virgin olive oils contain more antioxidants. 1 tablespoon olive oil serving contains less than 0 mg of phosphorus, less than a mg of potassium, and 1 mg of sodium.

Vitamins and minerals

Our bodies need vitamins to be able to function correctly. The best way to achieve this is make sure you eat a well-rounded diet. However, if you have chronic kidney disease, you may not be able to get all the recommended vitamins through diet alone. Vitamins that are usually recommended by your renal dietitian are vitamin C, biotin, pantothenic acid, niacin, vitamin B12, B6, B2, B1, and folic acid. You must consult your doctor or dietician before starting to take vitamin supplements.

EATING OUT AND SHOPPING ON A RENAL DIET

ADVICE FOR DINING OUT

You don't have to miss out on your favorite restaurant or cuisines. Look out for small or half portions and ask your server for your foods to be cooked without extra salts, butters or sauces. Avoid fried foods and opt for grilled or poached instead.

If you know you are going out to eat, plan ahead. Look at their menu beforehand and decide what you will order to avoid anxiety or stress on the night! Use the food lists above to help you choose and don't feel bad about asking them to cater for your needs. Be sure to take any phosphorus binders, if they have been prescribed to you. Take them will your meal instead of waiting until you get home.

ADVICE FOR TRAVELING

Whatever your travel plans, you will have to eat. If you plan ahead, you should be able to make a meal plan with your renal dietitian. Tell your dietitian where you are going and what you expect to eat at your destination.
Remember to pack any prescriptions you may have such as phosphate binders.
If you are diabetic remember to keep carbohydrates at a minimum. Try not to eat sweets like sweetened drinks, fruit juices, cakes, pies, and candy. Don't consume salty foods like chips, crackers, and pretzels. Also limit condiments such as soy sauce, salad dressing, and ketchup. Keep a check on your blood sugar daily.

If going on a road trip or camping, avoid processed meats. If at all possible, use fresh-cooked meats, low-sodium deli meats, unsalted chicken or tuna. Have unsalted pretzels or crackers instead of potato chips. Salty foods need to be avoided if you are on a fluid restricted diet. Take along nutritional drinks formulated for kidney patients. These can always be used as a meal replacement if need be. Remember to check for sodium content. Do not consume dairy products unless they are allowed as part of your diet plan.

If you are going on a cruise, all those buffet foods can be tempting to eat 24 hours a day. To help with this predicament try to select fruits, salads, and vegetables. Remember to include a good source of protein with every meal. Avoid breads and sauces that are salty. Let the cruise line know of your dietary needs, most are willing to prepare special foods for you. Low-sodium meals may also be available. Pack your own snacks to eat between meals.

If you are going to be traveling abroad and don't speak the language, bring a phrasebook that has a section for ordering food.

COOKING TIPS

1. Grill meats instead of frying.
2. Steam or boil vegetables instead of frying.
3. Use healthy oils such as extra virgin olive oil to shallow fry.
4. Soak fruit and vegetables in warm water for 2 hours before cooking in order to reduce potassium levels – especially potatoes!
5. When using canned beans and vegetables, make sure to rinse and drain them.
6. Drain liquid from canned or frozen vegetables of fruits.

KITCHEN EQUIPMENT:

In order to help you get started on this diet, there are a few things that you will need in order to be able to prepare the foods and meals in this cookbook:

- Blender/ food processor
- Crock pot, pots, skillet
- Steam basket/steamer/colander
- Oven dish, tray
- Potato masher
- Large mixing bowls
- Foil/cling film
- Tupperware boxes
- Stocking your cupboard:
- Ensure you purchase a variety of dry ingredients that can be used to add flavor to your foods (see foods to enjoy list).
- A 2 quart slow cooker for 2/4 quart slow cooker for families

ONE LAST THING:

Always remember to use new recipes and ingredients after speaking to your doctor or dietitian; your needs will be unique to you depending on the stage of chronic kidney disease you're experiencing. We hope that with your doctor's advice, along with our guidance and recipes, that you can continue to enjoy cooking, eating and sharing meal times with your love ones.

Please note:
it is crucial you see your dietitian to determine the levels you should be consuming each day and adjust the serving sizes according to your individual requirements if necessary.

All nutrition levels have been calculated using The US Department of Agriculture's Super Tracker website www.supertracker.usda.gov and may differ depending on specific brands. It is always advised to track your nutrition using a tracking site such as this one or by studying the individual labels on foods.

BREAKFAST

Mediterranean Omelet

SERVES 2 / PREP TIME: 2 MINUTES / COOK TIME: 10 MINUTES

Fresh herby omelet.

---

2 eggs
Pinch of black pepper
1 tbsp chopped chives
1 tsp chopped parsley
1/4 cup almond milk
1 tbsp extra virgin olive oil

1/2 red onion, peeled and thinly sliced
1 clove of garlic, crushed

---

1. Soak vegetables in water for up to 2 hours before cooking if possible.
2. Beat eggs, pepper, herbs and almond milk in a separate bowl.
3. Heat the oil in a skillet over a medium heat.
4. Add the onion and garlic to the skillet and sauté on medium heat for a few minutes until soft.
5. Pour the eggs evenly into the skillet and cook over a medium heat for 6-7minutes.
6. Use a spatula to gently lift the edge. If it comes away easily, shake the pan a little to loosen the omelet from the bottom.
7. Flip or fold in half and continue to cook for a further 2-3 minutes.
8. Slice in half and serve immediately.

Per Serving: Calories 186
Protein 7
Carbohydrates 7
Fat 7
Sodium 117
Potassium 124
Phosphorus 72

Egg & Spinach Muffins

SERVES 2 / PREP TIME: 10 MINUTES / COOK TIME: 25 MINUTES

So easy to prepare - just bung them in the oven!

1/3 cup green onions, washed diced
1 cup baby spinach leaves, washed
2 eggs
1 tsp sage, dried
1 tbsp almond milk
Pinch of black pepper
1 4 hole muffin tin

---

1. Preheat oven to 180°C/350°F/Gas Mark 4.
2. Line a 4 hole muffin tin with paper muffin wrappers or melted coconut oil.
3. Layer each muffin case with 1/4 green onions and spinach.
4. In a separate bowl, beat the eggs, herbs, almond milk and black pepper.
5. Pour 1/4 of the egg mixture into each muffin cup.
6. Leave a little gap at the top of each case.
7. Bake in the oven for 25 minutes, or until muffins have slightly risen and egg is cooked through.
8. Remove muffins from pan and serve hot.
9. Enjoy with a side salad if desired.

Per Serving: Calories 92
Protein 7 g
Carbohydrates 2 g
Fat 0 g
Sodium 155 mg
Potassium 188 mg
Phosphorus 28 mg

Lemon & Tarragon Crepes

SERVES 2 / PREP TIME: 5 MINUTES / COOK TIME: 4 MINUTES

Light and bubbling with a hint of herbs and citrus to cut through!

---

2 eggs
1 tbsp tarragon, stalks removed and
finely chopped
Pinch of black pepper
1-1/3 cups almond milk
3/4 cup all purpose white flour
1 tbsp coconut oil
1 lemon

---

1. Whisk eggs, tarragon, pepper and milk in a bowl.
2. Slowly sift in flour and whisk for 1 minute.
2. Heat a skillet over a medium to high heat.
3. Add coconut oil and allow to melt
4. Using a 1/4 cup measure, pour the batter evenly into the skillet.
5. Cook for 3-4 minutes until bubbling.
6. Loosen the edges of the crepe with a spatula and remove from the pan when golden on the bottom.
7. Repeat for the rest of the mixture.
8. Slice the lemon in half, squeeze over the crepes to serve.

Per Serving: Calories 408
Protein 15 g
Carbohydrates 60 g
Fat 10 g
Sodium 250 mg
Potassium 300 mg
Phosphorus 87 mg

Parsley Omelet

SERVES 2 / PREP TIME: 5 MINUTES / COOK TIME: 7 MINUTES

A slight twist on a traditional omelet.

1 tbsp canola oil
1/4 onion, diced
1/4 fresh green bell pepper, diced
1 egg
2 egg whites
2 tbsp almond milk
2 sprigs fresh parsley

1. Heat the oil in a skillet over a medium heat.
2. Add the diced onion and green pepper and sauté for 2 minutes.
3. Whisk the eggs and milk together.
4. Pour the eggs evenly across the vegetable mixture in the skillet.
5. Allow to cook for 5-6 minutes on a medium heat until cooked through.
6. Use your spatula to fold or flip and cook for a further minute.
7. Sprinkle with parsley and cut in half to serve.

Per Serving: Calories 154
Protein 10 g
Carbohydrates 8 g
Fat 9 g
Sodium 47 mg
Potassium 307 mg
Phosphorus 76 mg

Chili Scrambled Tortillas

SERVES 2 / PREP TIME: 5 MINUTES / COOK TIME: 5 MINUTES

Kick-start your morning with these fiery wraps.

non-stick cooking spray
2 egg whites
3 tbsp green chillis, diced
1/4 tsp ground cumin

1/2 tsp hot pepper sauce
2 flour tortillas

1. Spray a skillet with non-stick cooking spray and heat over a medium heat.
2. In a bowl, beat the eggs with the green chillis, cumin and hot sauce.
3. Pour egg mixture evenly into the skillet and cook for 1 to 2 minutes, stirring constantly until the eggs are cooked through.
4. Heat tortillas for 20 seconds in a microwave or in a separate dry skillet over a medium heat.
5. Top each tortilla with the scrambled eggs and roll.
6. Enjoy warm!

Per Serving: Calories 247
Protein 12 g
Carbohydrates 36 g
Fat 3 g
Sodium 77 mg
Potassium 199 mg
Phosphorus 119 mg

Speedy Beef & Bean Sprout Brekki

SERVES 5 / PREP TIME: 2 MINUTES / COOK TIME: 25 MINUTES

A protein and iron-rich breakfast which tastes delicious.

---

1 tbsp coconut oil for cooking
5 oz beef frying strips (organic grass-fed)
1/2 cup onions, finely diced
1 garlic clove, crushed
1 thumb-size piece of ginger, grated
1/2 cup bean sprouts
1 tbsp balsamic vinegar for dressing

---

1. Heat 1/2 the coconut oil in a large skillet over a high heat.
2. Add the beef frying strips and cook according to package directions.
3. Remove beef from the skillet and place to one side.
4. Add 1/2 coconut oil to the skillet and sauté the onions and garlic for 3-4 minutes over a medium heat until soft (don't brown!)
5. Now add the ginger and bean sprouts.
6. Serve 1/2 the vegetables on each serving dish and top with the beef strips.
7. Drizzle with balsamic vinegar to serve.

Per Serving: Calories 69
Protein 12 g
Carbohydrates 3 g
Fat 1 g
Sodium 35 mg
Potassium 25 mg
Phosphorus 44 mg

Chicken & Red Pepper Muffins

SERVES 4 / PREP TIME: 10 MINUTES / COOK TIME: 30 MINUTES

Fresh and revitalising breakfast muffins.

---

1 tbsp extra virgin olive oil
5 oz skinless chicken breasts, diced
1 red bell pepper, diced
1/2 cup spinach leaves, washed
2 English muffin
Pinch black pepper
1 tbsp fresh basil, finely chopped (optional)

---

1. Heat 1/2 the olive oil in a skillet over a medium to high heat.
2. Add the diced chicken and cook, turning occasionally for 20 minutes or according to package directions.
3. Ensure the chicken is cooked through by sticking a sharp knife into the centre (it should come out clean).
4. Remove from the pan and place to one side.
5. Now add the red pepper to the skillet and saute for 5-6 minutes or until soft.
6. Add the spinach to the skillet and turn off the heat (the spinach will wilt slightly).
7. Slice the English muffin in half and lightly toast in a toaster or under the grill.
8. Meanwhile, mix the rest of the olive oil with the chopped basil and pepper.
9. Top each half of the muffin with the chicken, followed by the vegetables and lastly drizzle with the basil oil.

Per Serving: Calories 139
Protein 10 g
Carbohydrates 14 g
Fat 6 g
Sodium 140 mg
Potassium 121 mg
Phosphorus 113 mg

Vegetarian Eggs Benedict

SERVES 4 / PREP TIME: 5 MINUTES / COOK TIME: 10 MINUTES

Delicious healthy version of a posh brunch!

2 English muffins
1 tsp balsamic vinegar
3 cups water
4 eggs
1/2 cup spinach leaves

1. Slice English muffins in half and toast them.
2. Add the vinegar and water into a pan.
3. Bring to a boil and then lower the heat.
4. Whilst stirring the water with a wooden spoon, crack the eggs into the water one at a time.
5. Cover and simmer for 3 to 5 minutes or 1-2 minutes longer if you like hard yolks.
6. Remove eggs with a slotted spoon and place on top of the English muffin halves; cover and keep warm.
7. Top with freshly washed spinach leaves, a drizzle of balsamic vinegar, and a sprinkle of black pepper.
8. Serve!

Per Serving: Calories 137
Protein 8 g
Carbohydrates 13 g
Fat 5 g
Sodium 176 mg
Potassium 174 mg
Phosphorus 126 mg

Chilli Tofu Scramble

SERVES 2 / PREP TIME: 5 MINUTES / COOK TIME: 10 MINUTES

Tofu soaks up the flavors of whatever it's cooked with so add some spice!

---

1 tsp coconut oil
1/2 cup green onions, finely diced
1 red chilli, de-seeded and finely diced
6oz tofu, drained
1/2 lime

---

1. Heat the oil in a skillet or wok over a medium to high heat.
2. Add the green onions and sauté for 1-2 minutes.
3. Add the chili and sauté for 1 minute.
4. Add the tofu and cook for 5-6 minutes or according to package directions.
5. Slice the lime in half, squeeze over the tofu and stir.
6. Enjoy.

Per Serving: Calories 272
Protein 15 g
Carbohydrates 15 g
Fat 20 g
Sodium 15 mg
Potassium 289 mg
Phosphorus 113 mg

Vanilla Pancakes (German Pancakes)

SERVES 4 / PREP TIME: 5 MINUTES / COOK TIME: 10 MINUTES

Sweet breakfast treat!

2/3 cup all-purpose flour
4 large eggs
1 cup unsweetened almond milk
1/4 tsp vanilla extract
non-stick cooking spray

1. Sift the flour into a mixing bowl.
2. Whisk the eggs into the flour.
3. Now add the milk and vanilla extract and beat until smooth.
4. Heat a non-stick skillet over a medium heat with non-stick cooking spray.
5. Pour 3 tablespoons of the batter into the skillet to cover.
6. Cook for 1 minute until the pancake is brown on the bottom.
7. Flip pancake and brown the other side.
8. Remove and keep warm.
9. Repeat until the batter is gone.
10. Serve with your choice of topping.

Per Serving: Calories 102
Protein 7 g
Carbohydrates 3 g
Fat 5 g
Sodium 161 mg
Potassium 165 mg
Phosphorus 140 mg

Renal-Friendly Rice Pudding

SERVES 4 / PREP TIME: 5 MINUTES / COOK TIME: 25 MINUTES

Wholesome and tasty!

---

2 cups water
2 cups rice milk
8 tbsp uncooked bulgur
1 cup canned apricots, drained
Pinch nutmeg

---

1. Heat the water and milk in a pot over a medium to high heat.
2. Bring to the boil and add the bulgur and apricots.
3. Lower the heat to a simmer, stirring occasionally for 20-25 minutes.
4. When the bulgur is soft, remove the pot from the heat and stir in the nutmeg.
5. Leave to stand for 5 minutes.
6. Stir through with a fork and serve.

Per Serving: Calories 119
Protein 5 g
Carbohydrates 26 g
Fat 1 g
Sodium 53 mg
Potassium 89 mg
Phosphorus 21 mg

Apple & Cinnamon Muffins

SERVES 6 / PREP TIME: 15 MINUTES / COOK TIME: 25 MINUTES

Treat yourself!

---

1 cup almond milk
1/2 tbsp apple cider vinegar
1 1/2 cups all-purpose flour
1/2 cup granulated sugar
1/4 tbsp baking soda (Ener-G substitu-
ate)
1/2 tsp ground cinnamon
1/4 cup canola oil
1 tbsp pure vanilla extract
6 hole muffin tin

1/2 cup apple sauce

---

1. Preheat oven to 190°C/375°F/Gas Mark 5.
2. Line the tin with paper cases.
3. In a bowl, stir the milk and vinegar and leave to rest for 5 minutes.
4. Meanwhile in a separate bowl, mix the flour, sugar, baking soda substitute, and cinnamon.
5. Now add the oil and the vanilla to the milk mixture from earlier and stir through thoroughly.
6. Now add the liquid mixture to the dry ingredients and stir until combined.
7. Fold through the apple sauce.
8. Spoon the mixture into the muffin cases and bake in the oven for 25 minutes or until golden and cooked through.
9. Stick a knife into the centre and it should come out clean.
10. Cool on a rack for 10 minutes before serving.

Per Serving: Calories 153
Protein 0 g
Carbohydrates 19 g
Fat 10 g
Sodium 270 mg
Potassium 72 mg
Phosphorus 47 mg

Homemade Turkey Patties

SERVES 4 / PREP TIME: 10 MINUTES / COOK TIME: 15 MINUTES

Patties are often unkind to our kidneys but these can be enjoyed guilt free!

---

1 tsp fennel seeds, crushed
6oz ground turkey,
1/8 tsp garlic powder
1/8 tsp onion powder

---

1. Crush the fennel seed using a pestle and mortar or blender.
2. In a bowl combine the turkey meat with the crushed fennel seeds, garlic powder, and onion powder.
3. Cover the bowl and refrigerate overnight if possible.
4. Divide the turkey into 4 portions and flatten using the palms of your hands into patties to cook.
5. Heat a non-stick skillet over a medium heat and add the patties until browned and cooked through (10-15 minutes).

Per Serving: Calories 69
Protein 7 g
Carbohydrates 1 g
Fat 3 g
Sodium 40 mg
Potassium 17 mg
Phosphorus 103 mg

Breakfast Smoothie

SERVES 4 /   PREP TIME: 5 MINUTES /   COOK TIME: NA

Packed with Vitamin C - this sweet and sour combination tastes amazing.

1/2 grapefruit, peeled and diced
6 cups water
1/2 cup canned papaya, drained

1. Add all ingredients to a blender or smoothie maker and blend until smooth.
2. Serve over ice.

Per Serving: Calories 18
Protein 4 g
Carbohydrates 15 g
Fat 20 g
Sodium 1 mg
Potassium 33 mg
Phosphorus 12 mg

Smoked Salmon & Dill Bagels

SERVES 2 / PREP TIME: 5 MINUTES / COOK TIME: 5 MINUTES

Omega-3 and delicious-this is a great Sunday morning breakfast.

1 tbsp honey
1/2 lemon
1 tsp dill, fresh or dried
1 bagel
4oz Smoked Salmon

1. Whisk the honey, lemon juice and dill together.
2. Slice the bagel in half and lightly toast.
3. Top with the salmon and squeeze the dressing over the top to serve.

Per Serving: Calories 215
Protein 15 g
Carbohydrates 30 g
Fat 3 g
Sodium 384 mg
Potassium 150 mg
Phosphorus 163 mg

Winter Berry Smoothie

SERVES 2 / PREP TIME: 5 MINUTES / COOK TIME: NA

Vibrant in color and vitamins alike.

1/4 cup blackberries
1/4 cup cherries, pitted
1/4 cup cranberries
2 cups water

1. Blend all ingredients until smooth in a blender or smoothie maker.
2. Serve right away.

Per Serving: Calories 21
Protein 2 g
Carbohydrates 5 g
Fat 0 g
Sodium 1 mg
Potassium 62 mg
Phosphorus 10 mg

Breakfast in a Pan

SERVES 4 / PREP TIME: 5 MINUTES / COOK TIME: 20 MINUTES

A One Pot Stop!

---

1 tbsp coconut oil
1 red bell pepper, diced
4 oz cooked skinless turkey breast
1/2 cup spinach leaves, washed
1 tsp oregano
1/4 cup scallions
2 egg whites, beaten

---

1. Preheat the broiler to a medium-high heat.
2. Into an oven proof skillet add the coconut oil over a medium heat until melted.
3. Add the pepper and turkey and sauté for 10-15 minutes until soft.
4. Now add the spinach, oregano and scallions and mix for 2 minutes.
5. Add the egg whites and mix together.
6. Place under the broiler for 4-5 minutes until the eggs are cooked.
7. Divide into 2 portions and serve.

Per Serving: Calories 91
Protein 11 g
Carbohydrates 2 g
Fat 3 g
Sodium 37 mg
Potassium 113 mg
Phosphorus 80 mg

Grilled Vegetables

SERVES 4 / PREP TIME: 5 MINUTES / COOK TIME: 15 MINUTES

Start your day with color!

1/4 green bell pepper, diced
1/4 red bell pepper, diced
1/4 yellow bell pepper, diced
1/4 zucchini, diced
1/4 red onion, diced
1 tbsp extra virgin olive oil
1 tsp thyme, fresh or dried
1 tsp oregano

---

1. Preheat the broiler to a medium-high heat.
2. Chop the vegetables into chunky pieces and if possible soak in warm water prior to use.
3. Add the vegetables, oil and herbs to an oven dish and toss with your hands.
4. Place under the broiler for 10-15 minutes or until vegetables are lightly grilled.
5. Serve alone or with your choice of salad.

Per Serving: Calories 43
Protein 0 g
Carbohydrates 2 g
Fat 3 g
Sodium 50 mg
Potassium 58 mg
Phosphorus 35 mg

Kidney Friendly Porridge

SERVES 2 / PREP TIME: 5 MINUTES / COOK TIME: 10 MINUTES

Warm & sweet!

---

1 cup water
1/2 cup cream of wheat farina
1/2 cup canned pears, drained and sliced
Pinch ground nutmeg

---

1. Bring the water to a boil in a saucepan.
2. Remove from the heat and add the cream of wheat slowly.
3. Stir continuously until combined.
4. Return to the heat once more and bring to the boil.
5. Lower the heat and cook for 3-4 minutes until thickened.
6. Stir through the canned pears and nutmeg.
7. Serve warm.

Per Serving: Calories 205
Protein 5 g
Carbohydrates 44 g
Fat 2 g
Sodium 3 mg
Potassium 92 mg
Phosphorus 18 mg

POULTRY

Grilled Spiced Turkey

SERVES 4 / PREP TIME: 5 MINUTES / COOK TIME: 20 MINUTES

So simple and succulent.

---

1 tbsp olive oil
1 tsp cinnamon
1 tsp nutmeg
1 tsp curry powder
6oz turkey breast, skinless and sliced

---

1. Whisk the oil and spices together and baste the turkey slices, coating thoroughly.
2. Cover and leave to marinade for as long as possible (ideally overnight).
3. When ready to cook, preheat the broiler to a medium-high heat and layer the turkey slices on a baking tray.
4. Place under the broiler for 15-20 minutes or according to package directions.
5. Turn occasionally.
6. Serve once cooked through with a side of vegetables or salad.

Per Serving: Calories 101
Protein 9 g
Carbohydrates 6 g
Fat 11 g
Sodium 42 mg
Potassium 27 mg
Phosphorus 102 mg

Herby Chicken Stew

SERVES 6 / PREP TIME: 5 MINUTES / COOK TIME: 40 MINUTES

Warming and hearty!

---

1 tsp olive oil
10 oz chicken breast, skinless and diced
1/2 cup eggplant, diced
1/2 red onion, diced
1 cup water
1 tsp oregano, fresh or dried
1 tsp thyme, fresh or dried
Pinch of black pepper
1/2 cup white rice

---

1. Soak vegetables in warm water prior to use if possible.
2. Heat an oven-proof pot over a medium-high heat and add olive oil.
3. Add the diced chicken breast and brown in the pot for 5-6 minutes, stirring to brown each side.
4. Once the chicken is browned, lower the heat to medium and add the vegetables to the pot to sauté for 5-6 minutes - careful not to let vegetables brown.
5. Add the water, herbs and pepper and bring to the boil.
6. Reduce the heat and simmer (lid on) for 30-40 minutes or until chicken is thoroughly cooked through.
7. Meanwhile, prepare your rice by rinsing in cold water first and then adding to a pan of cold water (1 cup) and bringing to the boil over a high heat.
8. Reduce the heat to medium and cook for 15 minutes.
9. Drain the rice and add back to the pan with the lid on to steam until the stew is ready.
10. Serve the stew on a bed of rice and enjoy!

Per Serving: Calories 143
Protein 15 g
Carbohydrates 9 g
Fat 5 g
Sodium 12 mg
Potassium 20 mg
Phosphorus 153 mg

Lemon & Herb Chicken Wraps

SERVES 4 / PREP TIME: 5 MINUTES / COOK TIME: 30 MINUTES

Delicious for a quick snack!

---

1 tbsp olive oil
1 lemon
2 tbsp fresh cilantro, finely chopped
Pinch of black pepper
4 oz chicken breasts, skinless and
sliced
1/2 red bell pepper, sliced
4 large iceberg lettuce leaves, washed
and sliced

---

1. Preheat the oven to 190°C/375°F/Gas Mark 5.
2. Mix the oil, juice of 1/2 lemon, cilantro and black pepper.
3. Marinate the chicken in the oil marinade, cover and leave in the fridge for as long as possible.
4. Wrap the chicken in parchment paper, drizzling over the remaining marinade.
5. Place in the oven in an oven dish for 25-30 minutes or until chicken is thoroughly cooked through and white inside.
6. Divide the sliced bell pepper and layer onto each lettuce leaf.
7. Divide the chicken onto each lettuce leaf and squeeze over the remaining lemon juice to taste.
8. Season with a little extra black pepper if desired.
9. Wrap and enjoy!

Per Serving: Calories 200
Protein 9 g
Carbohydrates 5 g
Fat 13 g
Sodium 25 mg
Potassium 125 mg
Phosphorus 196 mg

Carrot & Ginger Chicken Noodles

SERVES 4 / PREP TIME: 5 MINUTES / COOK TIME: 10 MINUTES

Fresh and revitalising!

---

1 tsp coconut oil
4 oz chicken breasts, skinless and
sliced
2 tsp fresh ginger, grated
1 garlic clove, minced
1 green onion, sliced
1 carrot, peeled and grated
1 lime
1 cup rice noodles, cooked

---

1. Heat a wok or large pan over a medium to high heat.
2. Add the coconut oil to a pan and once melted, add the sliced chicken and brown for 4-5 minutes.
3. Now add the ginger and garlic and sauté for 4-5 minutes.
4. Add the green onion, carrot and lime juice to the wok.
5. Add the cooked noodles to the wok and toss until hot through.
6. Serve piping hot and enjoy.

Per Serving: Calories 187
Protein 11 g
Carbohydrates 25 g
Fat 5 g
Sodium 39 mg
Potassium 91 mg
Phosphorus 178 mg

Marjoram Chicken & Cauliflower Rice

SERVES 4 / PREP TIME: 10 MINUTES / COOK TIME: 35 MINUTES

An exciting take on your usual bland chicken meals.

---

1 cup cauliflower
1 tsp olive oil
1/2 onion, finely diced
2 tsp marjoram
6oz chicken breast, skinless and sliced
Pinch of black pepper

---

1. Grate the cauliflower into rice-sized pieces (alternatively, use a food processor for 10 seconds to whiz up the cauliflower into small pieces).
2. Heat the oil in a wok or pan over a medium heat.
3. Sauté the onion in the wok for 4-5 minutes until it starts to soften.
4. Sprinkle 1 tsp of the marjoram over the onions to coat.
5. Add the chicken to the pan and sauté for 6-7 minutes to brown.
6. Continue to cook on a medium heat for 20-25 minutes.
7. Meanwhile, bring a pot of water (3 cups) to the boil over a high heat and add the cauliflower rice.
8. Add 1 tsp marjoram to the pot.
9. Turn down the heat immediately and cook the cauliflower for 5-6 minutes.
10. Drain and add the cauliflower to the wok with the chicken.
11. Stir and serve.

Per Serving: Calories 123
Protein 14 g
Carbohydrates 5 g
Fat 5 g
Sodium 17 mg
Potassium 125 mg
Phosphorus 125 mg

Chicken & Water Chestnut Noodles

SERVES 4 / PREP TIME: 5 MINUTES / COOK TIME: 25 MINUTES

Delicious for lunch or dinner.

2 tsp coconut oil
4oz skinless chicken breasts, sliced
2 cup rice noodles
1 garlic clove, crushed
1 carrot, grated
1/2 cup water chestnut, canned
1 lime, juiced

1. Heat 1 tsp oil on a medium heat in a skillet or wok.
2. Sauté the chicken breasts for about 15-20 minutes or until cooked through.
3. While cooking the chicken, place the noodles in a pot of boiling water for 5 minutes. Drain.
4. Add the garlic, carrots and water chestnuts to the wok and sauté for 3-4 minutes or until garlic aromas reach your nose!
5. Squeeze over the lime juice.
6. Serve hot straight away.

Per Serving: Calories 213
Protein 11 g
Carbohydrates 23 g
Fat 9 g
Sodium 27 mg
Potassium 4 mg
Phosphorus 99 mg

Turkey Kebabs & Red Onion Salsa

SERVES 8 / PREP TIME: 10 MINUTES /COOK TIME: 25 MINUTES

A leaner meat teamed with a chili salsa.

For the turkey:
1/2 lemon, juiced
2 garlic cloves, minced
1 tsp cumin
1 tsp turmeric
8oz turkey breasts, cut into cubes
8 metal kebab skewers
Lemon wedges to garnish

For the salsa:
1 red onion, diced
1 lemon, juiced
1 tsp white wine vinegar
1 tsp black pepper
1 tbsp olive oil
1 tsp of chilli flakes

---

1. Whisk the lemon juice, garlic, cumin and turmeric in a bowl to make your marinade.
2. Skewer the turkey cubes using kebab sticks (metal).
3. Baste the turkey on each side with the marinade, covering for as long as possible in the fridge or straight away if you're in a rush.
4. When ready to cook, preheat the oven to 400°F/200 °C/Gas Mark 6 and bake for 20-25 minutes or until turkey is thoroughly cooked through.
5. Prepare the salsa by mixing all the ingredients in a separate bowl.
6. Serve the turkey kebabs, garnished with the lemon wedges and the salsa on the side.

Per Serving: Calories 67
Protein 9 g
Carbohydrates 2 g
Fat 2 g
Sodium 1 mg
Potassium 25 mg
Phosphorus 75 mg

Griddled Chicken & Asparagus Linguine

SERVES 4 / PREP TIME: 5 MINUTES / COOK TIME:30 MINUTES

Light and fresh!

---

1 cup of asparagus stems
1 tsp extra virgin olive oil
4oz skinless chicken breast, diced
2 cups linguine pasta
1/2 lemon, juiced
1 tsp tarragon
Pinch of black pepper

---

1. Prepare asparagus stems by removing the hard part at the base (about a cm).
2. Heat a griddle pan on a medium to high heat and add the oil.
3. Add the diced chicken and sauté for 15-20 minutes or until thoroughly cooked through.
4. Meanwhile, cook your pasta in boiling water (4 cups) according to package directions.
5. Place to one side.
6. Wipe the griddle pan clean and place over the heat again.
7. Add the asparagus stems to the griddle pan for 5-10 minutes, turning to brown each side.
8. Drain the pasta and add the chicken to the pasta, heating until piping hot throughout.
9. Sprinkle with tarragon and black pepper and drizzle with a little lemon juice.
10. Top each portion with the asparagus stems.
11. Enjoy!

Per Serving: Calories 162
Protein 9 g
Carbohydrates 22 g
Fat 5 g
Sodium 85 mg
Potassium 67 mg
Phosphorus 134 mg

Herby Breaded Chicken

SERVES 4 / PREP TIME: 10 MINUTES / COOK TIME: 30 MINUTES

Delicious!

1/2 cup fresh basil
1 cup fresh watercress
1 tsp extra virgin olive oil
2 pita bread
2 egg whites
4oz chicken breasts, cut into strips

---

1. Preheat oven to 350°f/170°c/Gas Mark 4.
2. Add the pita bread, herbs and olive oil to a blender or pestle and mortar and blend into breadcrumbs.
3. Pour into a shallow bowl.
4. Whisk the egg whites in a separate shallow bowl.
5. Individually, dip the chicken strips into the egg whites and then straight into the breadcrumbs to coat each side. (Add a little water to the breadcrumb mixture if you find it doesn't stick well).
6. Place onto a baking sheet.
7. Bake for at least 30 minutes in the oven, or until the chicken is completely cooked through.
8. Serve the chicken with watercress or your choice of salad on the side.

Per Serving: Calories 151
Protein 12 g
Carbohydrates 18 g
Fat 5 g
Sodium 230 mg
Potassium 98 mg
Phosphorus 112 mg

Chicken & White Wine Casserole

SERVES 8 / PREP TIME: 10 MINUTES / COOK TIME: 40 MINUTES

What a treat!

8oz skinless, boneless chicken breasts
1/2 cup all-purpose flour
1 tsp black pepper
2 1/2 tbsp unsalted butter
1 tsp olive oil
1 medium onion, sliced

2 medium garlic cloves, sliced
3 tbsp fresh flat-leaf parsley, chopped
1/2 cup dry white wine
4 cups water
2 tbsp lemon juice

---

1. Dice the chicken breasts.
2. Add 1/2 cup flour and black pepper into a shallow dish (reserve 1 tsp flour).
3. Add the chicken into the flour and shake to coat.
4. Now, melt 1 tbsp of the butter in a large skillet over a medium-high heat.
5. Add 1 tsp of the olive oil to the skillet.
6. Add the floured chicken to the skillet and sauté for 10-15 minutes until browned.
7. Add the onions and sauté for 3 minutes, whilst stirring.
8. Add the garlic and sauté for 1 minute, whilst stirring.
9. Add the wine to the skillet and turn up the heat to full.
10. Bring to a boil and then turn down the heat and simmer until the liquid thickens, stirring occasionally.
11. Add the reserved tsp flour to the water and stir.
12. Now add this to the pan.
13. Bring back to the boil on a high heat and then turn down to simmer for 10 minutes or until sauce is thickened.
14. Ensure the chicken is thoroughly cooked through.
15. Remove from the heat and stir in remaining butter and lemon juice.
16. Serve right away.

Per Serving: Calories 108
Protein 5 g
Carbohydrates 2 g
Fat 7 g
Sodium 88 mg
Potassium 39 mg
Phosphorus 91 mg

Filling Fajitas

SERVES 4 / PREP TIME: 10 MINUTES / COOK TIME: 25 MINUTES

A healthy version of the takeaway favorite.

---

4 iceberg lettuce leaves
4 oz ground lean turkey
1/2 onion, finely diced
1 red bell pepper, finely diced
1 tsp paprika
1 tsp chili powder

1 Tsp olive oil

---

1. Carefully pull off the leaves from the lettuce and rinse.
2. Mix the rest of the ingredients in a bowl (reserve the oil).
3. Heat the oil in a skillet over a medium to high heat.
4. Add the turkey mixture to the pan and cook for 15-20 minutes or until cooked through.
5. Once cooked, remove from the pan and add to the centre of each lettuce leaf before wrapping fajita style!
6. Enjoy.

Per Serving: Calories 97
Protein 7 g
Carbohydrates 6 g
Fat 6 g
Sodium 83 mg
Potassium 139 mg
Phosphorus 82 mg

Cranberry Chicken & Red Cabbage

SERVES 4 / PREP TIME: 5 MINUTES / COOK TIME: 30 MINUTES

This is a filling and healthy treat!

1/2 cup cranberries
1 tbsp apple cider vinegar
1 tsp cinnamon
1 cup water
1 tbsp olive oil
4oz boneless, skinless, chicken breasts
1/2 cup red onion, diced
1 cup of red cabbage, boiled

---

1. In a saucepan, add the cranberries, vinegar, cinnamon and 1 cup water over a medium to high heat.
2. Bring to the boil and allow to simmer until the sauce thickens for 15-20 minutes.
3. Meanwhile, heat the oil in a large skillet over a medium heat.
4. Add the chicken breasts and cook for 4-5 minutes on each side.
5. Add the onion and sauté until translucent. Take care not to let it brown.
6. Lower the heat, cover and cook for 15–20 minutes or until chicken breasts are thoroughly cooked through.
7. Add the boiled cabbage to the pan for 5 minutes or until warmed through.
8. Serve with the cranberry sauce.

Per Serving: Calories 180
Protein 5 g
Carbohydrates 32 g
Fat 4 g
Sodium 99 mg
Potassium 90 mg
Phosphorus 90 mg

Caribbean Turkey

SERVES 6 / PREP TIME: 5 MINUTES / COOK TIME: 40 MINUTES

Brings you the taste of the Caribbean!

---

1 garlic clove, minced
1 tbsp coconut oil, melted
2 tsp curry powder
1 tbsp Jamaican spice blend
6oz skinless turkey breast, diced
1 cup white rice
1 lime

---

1. Preheat the oven to 350°f/170°c/Gas Mark 4.
2. Prepare the marinade by mixing garlic, coconut oil and spices together before pouring over the turkey.
3. Add the turkey to a baking dish and place in the oven for 35-40 minutes.
4. Meanwhile prepare your rice by bringing a pan of water (2 cups) to the boil.
5. Add rice and cover and simmer for 20 minutes.
6. Drain and cover the rice and return to the stove for 5 minutes.
7. When the turkey is cooked through, serve on a bed of rice and squeeze fresh lime juice over the top.
8. Enjoy.

Per Serving: Calories 149
Protein 10 g
Carbohydrates 16 g
Fat 3 g
Sodium 28 mg
Potassium 70 mg
Phosphorus 128 mg

Turkey Chili & Rice

SERVES 6 / PREP TIME: 5 MINUTES / COOK TIME: 30 MINUTES

Rustle this up in a flash and enjoy!

1 tbsp extra virgin olive oil
1 red onion, finely diced
1 garlic clove
1 red chili, finely diced
1 red bell pepper, finely diced
1 tsp curry powder
6oz lean ground turkey
1/4 cup water
2 cups white rice
2 green onions, sliced

2 tbsp freshly chopped cilantro

1. Heat the oil in a skillet on a medium to high heat.
2. Throw in the onions and garlic and sauté for 5-6 minutes until translucent but take care not to brown.
3. Add the red pepper, chili and curry powder.
4. Now add the turkey mince and stir to combine.
5. Cook on a medium heat for 5 minutes or until turkey has browned.
6. Now add 1/4 cup water, cover the pan and leave to simmer on a low to medium heat for 20 minutes or until turkey is cooked through.
7. Meanwhile add your rice to a pan of cold water (4 cups) and bring to the boil.
8. Turn down the heat and simmer for 15 minutes.
9. Drain the rice, return the lid and steam for 5 minutes.
10. Serve the turkey chili on a bed of rice and garnish with freshly chopped cilantro and sliced green onions.

Per Serving: Calories 288
Protein 6 g
Carbohydrates 47 g
Fat 6 g
Sodium 38 mg
Potassium 69 mg
Phosphorus 126 mg

Grilled Pineapple Chicken

SERVES 4 / PREP TIME: 10 MINUTES / COOK TIME: 20 MINUTES

Fruity and scrumptious.

1/2 iceberg lettuce or similar, washed
and sliced
2 radishes, washed and sliced
1/2 cucumber, sliced
1 tsp extra virgin olive oil
1 tsp apple cider vinegar
4oz chicken breast, skinless
Pinch of black pepper
1 tsp dried thyme
1/2 cup canned pineapple rings, juices
drained

---

1. Preheat the broiler to a medium-high heat.
2. Prepare your salad by combining lettuce, radish and cucumber. Cover and place in the fridge.
3. Whisk oil and vinegar in a dressing bowl and place to one side.
4. Preheat the broiler to a medium-high heat.
5. Slice the chicken breast meat into strips.
6. Place the chicken on a baking tray and sprinkle with black pepper and thyme.
7. Place under the broiler for 10 minutes on each side or until thoroughly cooked through.
8. Add the pineapple rings to the broiler 5 minutes before the chicken time is up.
9. Serve the chicken strips and pineapple on a bed of salad and drizzle with the dressing prepared earlier.

Per Serving: Calories 87
Protein 26 g
Carbohydrates 6 g
Fat 4 g
Sodium 87 mg
Potassium 20 mg
Phosphorus 94 mg

Lemon & Oregano Easy Cook Chicken

SERVES 6 / PREP TIME: 10 MINUTES / COOK TIME: 25 MINUTES

A citrus twist on your usual chicken dish.

1/4 cup lemon juice
1/4 cup water
2 tbsp extra virgin olive oil
1 tsp dried oregano
1 bay leaf
6oz boneless, skinless chicken breasts, diced

---

1. Combine lemon juice, water,, olive oil, oregano and bay leaf in a glass dish or zip lock bag.
2. Add chicken breasts, turn to coat, and marinate for at least 2 hours in the fridge.
3. When ready to cook, preheat the broiler or grill to a medium-high heat.
4. Broil or grill chicken on an oven dish for 10 minutes per side or until thoroughly cooked through - test with a sharp knife in the centre of the chicken breast to ensure that no liquid seeps out and the meat is white all the way through.
5. Enjoy with your choice of rice, salad or pasta.

Per Serving: Calories 69
Protein 5 g
Carbohydrates 1 g
Fat 5 g
Sodium 87 mg
Potassium 14 mg
Phosphorus 75 mg

Baked Turkey Breast & Eggplant

SERVES 4 / PREP TIME: 10 MINUTES / COOK TIME: 40 MINUTES

Incredible!

---

1 tbsp coconut oil
4oz boneless turkey breasts, sliced
1/2 eggplant, sliced into discs
2 tbsp olive oil
1/2 cup fresh cilantro, chopped
Pinch black pepper
1/4 cup low sodium chicken broth
1/4 cup arugula, washed

---

1. Preheat the oven to 350°f/170°c/Gas Mark 4.
2. Heat the coconut oil in a wok or skillet over a medium to high heat and sauté the sliced turkey breasts for 5 minutes or until browned.
3. Remove from the heat and place on a plate.
4. Layer a deep oven or lasagna dish with half the eggplant discs.
5. Drizzle over half the olive oil and half the herbs.
6. Layer half the turkey slices on the top and repeat with the rest of the eggplant, oil and herbs.
7. Sprinkle over black pepper.
8. Pour over the chicken broth and place in the oven for 20-30 minutes until turkey is completely cooked through and stock is bubbling.
9. Serve with a bed of arugula on the side.

Per Serving: Calories 138
Protein 9 g
Carbohydrates 0 g
Fat 11 g
Sodium 28 mg
Potassium 100 mg
Phosphorus 73 mg

Festive Cranberry Turkey Breasts

SERVES 4 / PREP TIME: 5 MINUTES / COOK TIME: 35 MINUTES

A Christmas treat that can be enjoyed all year round!

4oz turkey breasts
1 cup cranberries
1 tsp nutmeg
1 tsp cinnamon
1 tsp black pepper
1 cup water
1 tsp red wine vinegar

1. Preheat the broiler to a medium heat.
2. Slice the turkey breast.
3. Add to a lined baking tray and broil for 20-30 minutes or until cooked through.
4. Meanwhile, heat a pot on a medium-high heat and add the rest of the ingredients.
5. Allow to boil and then turn down the heat and simmer for 15 minutes or until reduced to a thick sauce.
6. Serve the turkey breasts once cooked with a helping of cranberry sauce and your choice of vegetables.

Per Serving: Calories 63
Protein 9 g
Carbohydrates 4g
Fat 11 g
Sodium 28 mg
Potassium 101 mg
Phosphorus 72 mg

Sweet and Sour Chicken

SERVES 2 / PREP TIME: 10 MINUTES / COOK TIME: 30 MINUTES

An oriental infused chicken dish.

---

1 tbsp coconut oil
6oz boneless, skinless chicken breasts, diced
1 garlic clove, minced
1 cup celery, sliced
1 green bell pepper, sliced
1 small onion, diced
1 cup reduced-sodium chicken broth
1/4 cup apple cider vinegar
1/2 cup canned pineapple chunks, juices drained
1 cup cooked white rice

---

1. Heat a wok or skillet over a medium to high heat and add coconut oil.
2. Add the chicken, garlic, celery, pepper and onions and sauté for 5 minutes.
3. Add the broth and vinegar.
4. Cover and simmer over low heat for 15 minutes.
5. Add the pineapple.
6. Cook for a further 10 minutes, stirring occasionally.
7. Ensure chicken is thoroughly cooked through.
8. Serve over rice.

Per Serving: Calories 108
Protein 7 g
Carbohydrates 13 g
Fat 2 g
Sodium 105 mg
Potassium 140 mg
Phosphorus 126 mg

Honey Mustard Grilled Chicken

SERVES 2 / PREP TIME: 10 MINUTES / COOK TIME: 30 MINUTES

Mustard and honey can be beneficial to those with CKD in many ways but should be limited according to your specific needs.

1 tbsp deli-style mustard
1 tbsp honey
1 tsp apple cider vinegar
2 green onions, chopped
4oz boneless, skinless chicken breasts,
sliced

1. In a small bowl, combine the mustard, honey, vinegar and green onions to make a marinade and place to one side.
2. Reserve 1/4 cup of the marinade to serve with the cooked chicken.
3. Preheat the broiler or grill to a medium-high heat.
4. Grill the chicken strips on an oven dish for 5 minutes.
5. Brush with the marinade and turn several times until the chicken is thoroughly cooked through (approximately 15-20 minutes).
6. Remove from the grill and serve with the rest of the honey-mustard sauce.
7. Serve with a side of vegetables!

Per Serving: Calories 80
Protein 10 g
Carbohydrates 7 g
Fat 1 g
Sodium 172 mg
Potassium 25 mg
Phosphorus 156 mg

MEAT

Healthy Roast Dinner

SERVES 4 / PREP TIME: MARINATE AS LONG AS POSSIBLE / COOK TIME: 45 MINUTES

Rich in iron and B vitamins.

---

1 tbsp thyme
1 tbsp olive oil
1 tsp pepper
10 oz of lean rump steak
1 onion, peeled and sliced
4 turnips, peeled and diced
2 garlic cloves
1/4 cup fresh parsley, chopped

---

1. Preheat the oven to 450°f/250°c/Gas Mark 8.
2. Meanwhile, mix the thyme and black pepper with the olive oil.
3. Coat the rump steak and allow to marinate for as long as possible.
4. Add the rump steak to a shallow oven-proof dish and heat the hob to a high heat.
5. Sear each side of the beef steak for a few minutes until browned. If the baking dish is not suitable to place on the hob, do this in a separate skillet first.
6. Now add the vegetables and whole garlic cloves (skin on) to the baking dish (if your beef is already in the dish make sure you use tongs to lift it first).
7. Add the dish to the oven for 25 minutes before turning the heat down to 300°f/150°c/Gas Mark 2.
8. Continue to cook for a further 8 minutes and then remove and allow to rest (the beef will continue to cook in the resting time).
9. After 5 minutes, slice the steak with a carving knife and serve on top of the juicy vegetables. The garlic should be deliciously soft by now so serve this up too!
10. Garnish with fresh parsley.

Per Serving: Calories 183
Protein 20 g
Carbohydrates 6 g
Fat 8 g
Sodium 110 mg
Potassium 382 mg
Phosphorus 214 mg

Mini Burgers

SERVES 2 / PREP TIME: 5 MINUTES / COOK TIME: 20 MINUTES

Enjoy a treat now and then!

---

5 oz lean 100% grass-fed ground beef
1 egg white
1 tsp black pepper
1 tsp paprika
1 green onion, chopped
2 hamburger buns
1/4 cup arugula

---

1. Preheat the broiler/grill to a medium-high heat.
2. Mix the ground beef with the herbs, egg white, spices and green onions.
3. Use your hands to form 2 patties (about 1 inch thick).
4. Add to an oven proof baking tray and broil for 15 minutes or until meat is thoroughly cooked through. Use a knife to insert into the centre - the juices should run clear.
5. Slice your burger buns and stack with the burger and arugula.

Per Serving: Calories 227
Protein 17 g
Carbohydrates 23 g
Fat 7 g
Sodium 295 mg
Potassium 78 mg
Phosphorus 193 mg

Slow-Cooked Beef Stew

SERVES 4 / PREP TIME: 10 MINUTES / COOK TIME OVERNIGHT

Stick this in the slow cooker for succulent and tender meat.

1 tbsp of extra virgin olive oil
10 oz lean beef, cubed
1 onion, diced
1 red bell pepper, roughly chopped
1 tsp cumin
1 tsp turmeric
1 tsp curry powder
1 tsp oregano
1 bay leaf
4 cups of water
1/2 cauliflower, chopped and par-boiled

1. Heat the olive oil in a skillet over a medium to high heat.
2. Add the beef and cook for 5 minutes or until browned on each side.
3. Add the onion and pepper to the slow cooker and pour in the water.
4. Now add the herbs, spices and bay leaf. Pour in the water and stir.
5. Then cover the slow cooker and cook for at least 8 hours or overnight.
6. 10 minutes before the end, add the cauliflower.
7. Plate up and serve when ready to eat!

Per Serving: Calories 227
Protein 19 g
Carbohydrates 10 g
Fat 12 g
Sodium 72 mg
Potassium 313 mg
Phosphorus 193 mg

Parsley Pork Meatballs

SERVES 2 / PREP TIME: 5 MINUTES / COOK TIME: 30 MINUTES

Succulent pork meatballs with a garlic and olive oil sauce.

---

6 oz lean pork mince
2 tbsp extra virgin olive oil
1 garlic clove, crushed
1 tsp dried sage
1/2 red onion, finely chopped
For the herb oil:
1 tbsp extra virgin olive oil
1 garlic clove crushed
1/4 cup fresh parsley

---

1. Mix the mince, 1 tbsp oil, 1 garlic clove, onion and sage in a bowl.
2. Season with a little black pepper and separate into 8 balls, rolling with the palms of your hands.
3. Heat 1 tbsp oil in a pan over a medium heat and add the meatballs for 5 minutes or until browned.
4. Cover and lower heat to simmer for 15 minutes.
5. Mix 1 tbsp olive oil, garlic and parsley in a separate bowl to form your herb oil and place to one side.
6. Once meatballs are thoroughly cooked through, drizzle with the herb oil and serve.
7. A bed of arugula tastes great with these meatballs!

Per Serving: Calories 290
Protein 17 g
Carbohydrates 2 g
Fat 24 g
Sodium 5 mg
Potassium 53 mg
Phosphorus 44 mg

Ginger & Bean Sprout Steak Stir-Fry

SERVES 2 / PREP TIME: 4 MINUTES / COOK TIME: 10 MINUTES

Chinese inspired dish.

5oz lean organic beef steak, cut into
strips
1 tsp coconut oil
1/4 cup bean sprouts
1 green onion, finely sliced
2 tsp fresh ginger, grated
1 garlic clove, minced
1 tsp nutmeg

---

1. Slice the beef into strips and add to a dry hot pan, cooking for 4-5 minutes on each side or until cooked to your liking.
2. Place to one side.
3. Add the oil to a clean pan and sauté the bean sprouts and onions with the ginger, garlic and nutmeg for 1 minute.
4. Serve the beef strips on a bed of the vegetables and enjoy.

Per Serving: Calories 227
Protein 13 g
Carbohydrates 13 g
Fat 23 g
Sodium 50 mg
Potassium 258 mg
Phosphorus 170 mg

Lime & Chili Beef Tortilla

SERVES 2 / PREP TIME: 5 MINUTES / COOK TIME: 20 MINUTES

Fresh and filling.

---

1 tbsp coconut oil
1 lime
1 tsp chili flakes
1 garlic clove, minced
5 oz lean beef mince
1/2 green bell pepper, sliced
1/4 cup green onions, chopped
1 tortilla

---

1. Into a blender or pestle and mortar, add half the oil, lime juice, chili flakes and garlic and blitz until nearly smooth.
1. Heat the rest of the oil in a skillet or wok over a medium to high heat.
2. Add the beef mince and brown for 4 minutes.
3. Now add the green pepper and continue to cook for a further 10 minutes.
4. Add the green onions and marinade and mix through.
5. Preheat the broiler or grill to a medium high heat.
6. Slice the tortilla and place under the broiler until crispy.
7. Serve the beef chilli with the tortilla chips on top.
8. Enjoy!

Per Serving: Calories 243
Protein 18 g
Carbohydrates 16 g
Fat 12 g
Sodium 46 mg
Potassium 442 mg
Phosphorus 208 mg

Nutmeg Pork Loin With White Cabbage

SERVES 2 / PREP TIME: 5 MINUTES / COOK TIME: 20 MINUTES

Enjoy a taste of Germany!

2x 3oz lean pork loins
1 tsp nutmeg
Pinch black pepper
1 tbsp white wine vinegar
1/2 white cabbage, sliced
2 carrots, peeled and sliced

---

1. Preheat the broiler to a medium high heat.
2. Sprinkle the pork with nutmeg on both sides.
3. Add the pork loins to a baking tray and place under the broiler for 10-15 minutes or according to package guidelines.
4. Meanwhile, place a pot of water over a medium-high heat.
5. Add the pepper and vinegar to the pan.
6. Now add the cabbage and carrots for 5-10 minutes or until soft (make sure the water covers the vegetables).
7. Drain the cabbage and carrots and serve with the pork.
8. Enjoy!

Per Serving: Calories 97
Protein 13 g
Carbohydrates 7 g
Fat 2 g
Sodium 64 mg
Potassium 392 mg
Phosphorus 170 mg

Beef & Eggplant Lasagna

SERVES 4 / PREP TIME: 10 MINUTES / COOK TIME: 50 MINUTES

Creamy white sauce and succulent beef lasagna.

---

1 garlic clove, minced
1 onion, diced
12 oz lean ground beef
1 tsp cayenne pepper
1 tsp parsley
1 tsp black pepper
1 eggplant, sliced vertically

For the white sauce:
1 tbsp unsalted butter
1/4 cup plain flour
3/4 cup rice milk
1 tsp black pepper

---

1. Preheat the oven to 350°f/170°c/Gas Mark 4.
2. To prepare the beef: Heat a skillet on a medium to high heat and spray with cooking spray.
3. Add the onions and garlic for 5 minutes until soft.
4. Add the lean beef mince, season with herbs and spices, add water and cook for 10-15 minutes or until completely browned.
5. Meanwhile prepare the white sauce:
6. Heat a saucepan on a medium heat.
7. Add the butter to the pan on the side nearest to the handle.
8. Tilt the pan towards you and allow the butter to melt, whilst trying not to let it cover the rest of the pan.
9. Now add the flour to the opposite side of the pan and gradually mix the flour into the butter - continue to mix until smooth.
10. Add the milk and mix thoroughly for 10 minutes until lumps dissolve.
11. Add pepper.
12. Turn off the heat and place to one side.
13. Layer an oven proof lasagna dish with 1/3 eggplant slices.
14. Add 1/3 beef mince on top.
15. Layer with 1/3 white sauce.
16. Repeat for 2 more layers.
17. Cover and add to the oven for 25-30 minutes or until golden and bubbly.
18. Remove and serve piping hot!

Per Serving: Calories 223
Protein 16 g
Carbohydrates 16 g
Fat 11 g
Sodium 52 mg
Potassium 324 mg
Phosphorus 161 mg

Chili Beef Strips & Pineapple Salsa

SERVES 4 / PREP TIME: 5 MINUTES / COOK TIME: 15 MINUTES

Spice things up in the kitchen.

2 tbsp extra virgin olive oil	for the salsa:
1/2 red onion, diced	1/2 red onion, finely diced
1/2 red bell pepper, diced	1/2 lime, juiced
1 garlic clove, minced	1 tbsp fresh cilantro
1 red chili, finely diced	1/4 cup canned pineapple, diced
6 oz lean beef, cut into strips	2 cups cooked white rice

1. Add 1 tbsp oil to a hot pan or skillet over a medium-high heat.
2. Add onion, pepper, garlic and chili and sauté for 5 minutes until soft.
3. Add the beef to the pan and stir until browned.
4. Cook for a further 5-10 minutes or until beef is cooked through.
5. Prepare the salsa by mixing the salsa ingredients.
6. Serve the beef strips on a bed of rice with the pineapple salsa.

Per Serving: Calories 417
Protein 18 g
Carbohydrates 58 g
Fat 10 g
Sodium 27 mg
Potassium 313 mg
Phosphorus 123 mg

Beef & Ginger Noodles

SERVES 4 / PREP TIME: 5 MINUTES / COOK TIME: 15 MINUTES

A delicious wok-cooked meal.

---

1 cup rice noodles
1 tsp coconut oil
6 oz lean frying beef, cut into strips
1 garlic clove, minced
1 tbsp ginger, minced
1 tsp Chinese 5 spice
1/4 cup water chestnuts
1/4 cup green onions, diced

---

1. Prepare the noodles according to package guidelines.
2. Meanwhile, heat the oil in a wok or skillet over a high heat.
3. Sauté the beef for 5-10 minutes, turning once to brown each side.
4. Add the garlic and ginger to the pan and sauté for a 2-3 minutes until aromas are released.
5. Now add the spices and water chestnuts and sauté over a medium heat for 15 minutes or until the beef is soft.
6. Serve the beef over the noodles and sprinkle with the green onions.
7. Enjoy!

Per Serving: Calories 215
Protein 18 g
Carbohydrates 31 g
Fat 6 g
Sodium 137 mg
Potassium 308 mg
Phosphorus 106 mg

Apricot & Lamb Stew

SERVES 2 / PREP TIME: 5 MINUTES / COOK TIME: 1 HOUR & 15 MINUTES
Supreme!

1 tbsp of olive oil
4oz lean lamb fillets, cubed
1 onion, chopped
2 carrots, diced
1 cup of low sodium chicken broth

1 tsp dried rosemary
3 cups water
1/2 cup canned apricots, juices drained
1 tsp of chopped parsley

1. In a large casserole dish, heat the olive oil on a medium-high heat.
2. Add the lamb and cook for 5 minutes until browned.
3. Add the chopped onion and carrots.
4. Leave to cook for another 5 minutes until the vegetables begin to soften.
5. Add the chicken broth and rosemary.
6. Then cover the casserole and leave to simmer on a low heat for 1 hour until the lamb is tender and fully cooked through.
7. Add the apricots 20 minutes before serving time.
8. Plate up and serve with the chopped parsley to garnish.
9. Hint: You can do this in a pan and then transfer to a slow cooker to leave overnight if you prefer!

Per Serving: Calories 118
Protein 8 g
Carbohydrates 13 g
Fat 5 g
Sodium 180 mg
Potassium 254 mg
Phosphorus 157 mg

Beef And Turnip Stroganoff

SERVES 2 / PREP TIME: 10 MINUTES / COOK TIME: 4-5 HOURS IN CROCK POT

A kidney-friendly take on the classic!

---

1 tbsp black pepper
1 tsp dried oregano
1 garlic clove, minced
1/2 onion, diced
2 turnips, peeled and diced
1 cup low salt chicken or vegetable stock
1 cup water
4 oz stewing beef, diced
1/2 cup almond milk
1/4 cup plain flour

1 cup white rice
1/4 cup fresh parsley, chopped

---

1. In a crock-pot or slow cooker, add the pepper, oregano, garlic, onion, turnips, stock, water and beef.
2. Cover and cook on high for 4-5 hours or until beef is tender.
3. Add the flour and almond milk to the crock pot and mix until smooth.
4. Leave for 4-5 hours on HIGH.
5. When ready to serve, bring a pan of water (2 cups) to the boil and add the rice for 20 minutes.
6. Drain the water from the rice, add the lid and steam for 5 minutes.
7. Serve the rice with the creamy beef over the top and garnish with the fresh parsley.

Per Serving: Calories 487
Protein 23 g
Carbohydrates 68 g
Fat 13 g
Sodium 126 mg
Potassium 351 mg
Phosphorus 225 mg

Lamb Pita With Beets & Arugula

SERVES 2 / PREP TIME: 10 MINUTES / COOK TIME: 20 MINUTES

Moroccan spiced lamb burgers.

---

6 oz lean ground lamb
1/2 red onion, finely diced
1 tbsp parsley
1 tbsp extra virgin olive oil
1 clove of garlic, minced
1 tsp cumin
1/2 cup canned beets, juices drained
1 lemon, juiced
1 cup arugula
1/4 cucumber, sliced
2 pitta breads

---

1. Preheat the broiler on a medium to high heat.
2. Mix together the ground lamb, red onion, parsley, olive oil, garlic and cumin until combined.
3. Shape 1 inch thick patties using wet hands.
4. Add the patties to a baking tray and place under the broiler for 7-8 minutes on each side or until thoroughly cooked through.
5. Slice the beets and drizzle with lemon juice.
6. Mix the beets with the arugula and cucumber.
7. Lightly toast the pita breads and cut a slice to form a pocket.
8. Fill with the lamb burger patty and a portion of the beet salad.
9. Enjoy!

Per Serving: Calories 434
Protein 18 g
Carbohydrates 40 g
Fat 21 g
Sodium 115 mg
Potassium 248 mg
Phosphorus 212 mg

Pulled Pork & Apple Compote

SERVES 5 / PREP TIME: 15 MINUTES / COOK TIME: 4 HOURS

Mouthwatering!

---

1 tbsp extra virgin olive oil
10 oz boneless pork shoulder roast
1 onion, sliced
3 cloves garlic
1 cup water
3 tbsp red wine vinegar
1 tsp black pepper
2 cups cooking apples, peeled and chopped
2 tbsp brown sugar

1 tbsp nutmeg
3 cups of cooked white rice

---

1. Preheat oven to 350°f/180°c/Gas Mark 5.
2. Heat the oil in a skillet over a medium-high heat.
3. Add the pork shoulder and brown each side.
4. Add the pork with the onions and garlic to a baking dish, along with the water, red wine vinegar and black pepper.
5. Cover and bake for 3-4 hours or until pork is tender.
6. Now remove the cover and cook for a further 30 minutes.
7. Meanwhile, add the apples, nutmeg and brown sugar to a pan over a high heat and cover with water.
8. Leave to simmer for 15-20 minutes or until apples are soft.
9. Remove the pork from the oven and allow to cool before shredding the meat with a knife and fork.
10. Blend the apples in a food processor until smooth and dollop over a portion of the shredded meat to serve.
11. Enjoy with rice!

Per Serving: Calories 508
Protein 15 g
Carbohydrates 65 g
Fat 13 g
Sodium 60 mg
Potassium 289 mg
Phosphorus 260 mg

Spiced Lamb & Eggplant Curry

SERVES 4 / PREP TIME: 10 MINUTES / COOK TIME: 1 HOUR

Scrumptious lamb dish.

---

1 tsp olive oil
1 onion, diced
8 oz lean lamb steaks, cubed
1 cup almond milk (unenriched)
1 tsp curry powder
1 cup eggplant, roughly chopped

1 tbsp cilantro
4 pita breads

---

1. Heat the oil in a large pan over a medium-high heat and sauté the onions for 5 minutes or until soft.
2. Add the lamb for 5-10 minutes, turning to brown each side, before adding the milk and curry powder.
3. Bring to the boil, then turn down the heat and add the eggplant to the curry.
4. Cover and simmer for 45-50 minutes or until the lamb is soft and cooked through (top up with a little water if the curry starts to dry up).
5. Scatter with cilantro and serve with pita bread to mop up all of the lovely juices!
6. Hint: This can also be prepared in a slow cooker in the same way - just transfer the ingredients and leave overnight on LOW.

Per Serving: Calories 274
Protein 12 g
Carbohydrates 41 g
Fat 8 g
Sodium 300 mg
Potassium 268 mg
Phosphorus 197 mg

Sausage Meat & Fennel Pasta

SERVES 4 / PREP TIME: 5 MINUTES / COOK TIME: 25 MINUTES

Tomato-less but tasty pasta dish!

---

1 tbsp fennel seeds, ground
8oz lean ground pork
2 tbsp extra virgin olive oil
1/2 onion, diced
1/2 cup water
2 cups pasta
1 tsp fresh tarragon
1 tsp black pepper

---

1. Mix the ground fennel seeds with the pork mince.
2. Over a medium heat, add 1 tbsp oil to a pan and sauté the onions for 5 minutes or until soft.
3. Add the pork mince to the pan and brown for 5 minutes.
4. Add the water and leave the pork on a medium heat to simmer.
5. Now add the pasta to a pot of boiling water (4 cups) over a high heat and cook for 15 minutes or according to package directions.
6. Drain the pasta and stir into the pan of pork mince.
7. Add the fresh tarragon and 1 tbsp olive oil to the pasta and mix to combine.
8. Serve right away with a pinch of black pepper.

Per Serving: Calories 318
Protein 13 g
Carbohydrates 23 g
Fat 19 g
Sodium 37 mg
Potassium 200 mg
Phosphorus 152 mg

Red Thai Curry

SERVES 4 / PREP TIME: 10 MINUTES / COOK TIME: 50 MINUTES

A sensational lamb curry.

---

1 tbsp fresh basil leaves
1 red chili, diced
1 red bell pepper, diced
1/2 stick lemon grass, chopped
1 tbsp coconut oil
7oz lean lamb, cubed
1/2 white onion, diced
1 garlic clove, minced
1/2 cup almond/rice milk
1/2 cup water
2 cups cooked white rice

---

1. Blend the chili, red pepper, basil, lemon grass and oil in a blender until a paste is formed. Alternatively use a pestle and mortar.
2. Heat a wok or skillet over a medium to high heat.
3. Spray a little cooking spray into the pan and add the lamb breasts for 5 minutes on each side or until brown.
4. Add the onions and garlic and sauté for 3 minutes.
5. Now pour the rice milk, stock and paste into the pan and stir until dissolved.
6. Allow to simmer on a medium to low heat for 30-40 minutes or until lamb is soft.
7. Serve with the rice.

Per Serving: Calories 425
Protein 11 g
Carbohydrates 56 g
Fat 15 g
Sodium 68 mg
Potassium 248 mg
Phosphorus 262 mg

Pork Chops & Rainbow Salad

SERVES 2 / PREP TIME: 10 MINUTES / COOK TIME: OVERNIGHT

So simple yet so delicious!

---

1 tsp black pepper
1 tsp smoked paprika
2x 3oz pork chops, fat trimmed
1/4 cup scallions, sliced
1/4 red bell pepper, diced
1/4 green bell pepper, diced
1/4 cup corn
1 tsp dried tarragon
1 tbsp olive oil

---

1. Preheat the broiler or grill to a medium-high heat.
2. Sprinkle the black pepper and paprika over the pork chops and rub.
3. Broil or grill the chops for 10-12 minutes or according to package directions.
4. Meanwhile, mix the vegetables with the oil and tarragon.
5. Serve the pork chops with the rainbow salad on the side.

Per Serving: Calories 298
Protein 22 g
Carbohydrates 8 g
Fat 19 g
Sodium 196 mg
Potassium 410 mg
Phosphorus 225 mg

Rutabaga & Turnip Cottage Pie

SERVES 6/ PREP TIME: 10 MINUTES / COOK TIME: 1 HOUR

A kidney friendly version of the British staple.

---

1 cup rutabaga, peeled & sliced
1 turnip, peeled and sliced
1 tsp olive oil
1 onion, diced
2 carrots, peeled & diced
12 oz lean ground beef
1 tsp black pepper

---

1. Preheat the oven to 350°f/170°c/Gas Mark 4.
2. Bring a pot of water to the boil (3 cups) and add the rutabaga.
3. Turn down the heat slightly and allow to simmer for 20 minutes.
4. Add the turnip to this pan in the last 10 minutes.
5. Meanwhile, add the oil to a pan on a medium heat.
6. Add the onions and sauté for 4-5 minutes or until soft.
7. Now add the carrots and sauté for a further 5 minutes.
8. Add the ground beef and mix until beef is browned.
9. Add the water, turn the heat to high until it starts to bubble and then reduce the heat and add the black pepper.
10. Remove from the heat and check that the rutabaga and turnips are soft with a fork.
11. Drain and mash with a potato masher.
12. Pour the beef mixture into a rectangular oven dish.
13. Top with the mash.
14. Use your fork to gently score the top of the mash, creating soft lines along the top.
15. Add to the oven for 30-40 minutes or until golden brown.
16. Remove and serve immediately!

Per Serving: Calories 132
Protein 12 g
Carbohydrates 7 g
Fat 6 g
Sodium 62 mg
Potassium 409 mg
Phosphorus 134 mg

Egg Fried Rice & Beef

SERVES 4 / PREP TIME: 5 MINUTES / COOK TIME: 10-15 MINUTES

Ready in a flash!

---

1 tbsp coconut oil
8oz lean beef strips
1/4 cup cauliflower florets, thinly
sliced
1 cup cooked white rice
2 egg whites
1/4 cup scallions, sliced
Pinch black pepper

---

1. Heat the oil in a wok or pan over a medium-high heat.
2. Add the beef strips and cook, turning only once half way through for 8-10 minutes or depending on package guidelines.
3. Add the cauliflower slices to the pan and sauté for 3-4 minutes.
4. Remove the beef and cauliflower and place to one side.
5. Now add the rice to the wok and lower the heat.
6. Quickly, stir in the egg whites until combined with the rice.
7. Serve the beef and cauliflower on a bed of rice.
8. Scatter the scallions over the top.
9. Add black pepper to taste.

Per Serving: Calories 207
Protein 25 g
Carbohydrates 12 g
Fat 25 g
Sodium 64 mg
Potassium 254 mg
Phosphorus 162 mg

VEGETARIAN & VEGAN

Thai Tofu Broth

SERVES 4 / PREP TIME: 5 MINUTES / COOK TIME: 15 MINUTES

Tasty tofu with Thai flavors.

---

1 tbsp coconut oil
6oz drained, pressed and cubed tofu
1/2 onion, sliced
1/2 cup rice milk
1/2 cup water
1 cup rice noodles
1/2 chili, finely sliced
1/2 cup canned water chestnuts
1 cup of snow peas
1 tbsp lime juice
1/4 cup scallions, sliced

---

1. Heat the oil in a wok on a high heat and then sauté the tofu until brown on each side.
2. Add the onion and sauté for 2-3 minutes.
3. Add the rice milk and water to the wok until bubbling.
4. Lower to a medium heat and add the noodles, chili and water chestnuts.
5. Allow to simmer for 10-15 minutes and then add the snow peas for 5 minutes.
6. Serve with a sprinkle of scallions.

Per Serving: Calories 304
Protein 9 g
Carbohydrates 38 g
Fat 13 g
Sodium 36 mg
Potassium 114 mg
Phosphorus 101 mg

Succulent Vegan Burgers

SERVES 2 / PREP TIME: 5 MINUTES / COOK TIME: 20 MINUTES

The hot spicy salsa compliments the tempeh wonderfully.

---

2 slices of extra firm tempeh 2.5 oz
each
2 tbsp extra virgin olive oil
1 tsp dried oregano
1/2 cucumber, finely diced
1/4 red chili, finely diced
1/2 lime, juiced
1/4 red onion, finely diced
1/2 cup baby spinach
2 white buns

---

1. Marinate the tempeh in 1 tbsp oil and oregano combined.
2. Soak the vegetables in warm water prior to use and heat the broiler on a medium to high heat.
3. Prepare your cucumber salsa by mixing the cucumber with the red chili and lime juice.
4. Heat 1 tbsp olive oil in a skillet on a medium heat.
5. Sauté the onion in the skillet for 6-7 minutes or until caramelized.
6. Stir in the baby spinach for a further 3-4 minutes.
7. Place to one side.
8. Broil the tempeh on a lined baking tray for 4 minutes on each side.
9. Add the tempeh to the bun and top with caramelized onion and spinach.
10. Serve immediately with the cucumber salsa on the side.

Per Serving: Calories 406
Protein 16 g
Carbohydrates 389g
Fat 18 g
Sodium 274 mg
Potassium 68 mg
Phosphorus 72 mg

Delicious Vegetarian Lasagna

SERVES 4 / PREP TIME: 10 MINUTES / COOK TIME: 1 HOUR

Tastes just as good without the meat!

1/2 zucchini , sliced
1/2 red pepper, sliced
1 cup eggplant, sliced
1 cup of rice milk
1/2 pack of soft tofu
1 tbsp olive oil
1/2 red onion, diced
1 garlic clove, minced
1 tsp oregano
1 tsp basil
Pinch of black pepper to taste
3 lasagna sheets

---

1. Preheat oven to 325°F/170 °C/Gas Mark 3.
2. Slice zucchini, eggplant and pepper into vertical strips.
3. Add the rice milk and tofu to a food processor and blitz until smooth. Place to one side.
4. Heat the oil in a skillet over a medium heat and add the onions and garlic for 3-4 minutes or until soft.
5. Sprinkle in the herbs and pepper and allow to stir through for 5-6 minutes until hot.
6. Into a lasagne or suitable oven dish, layer 1 lasagna sheet, then 1/3 the eggplant, followed by 1/3 zucchini, then 1/3 pepper before pouring over 1/3 of tofu white sauce.
7. Repeat for the next 2 layers, finishing with the white sauce.
8. Add to the oven for 40-50 minutes or until veg is soft and can easily by sliced into servings.

Per Serving: Calories 235
Protein 5 g
Carbohydrates 10g
Fat 9 g
Sodium 35 mg
Potassium 129 mg
Phosphorus 66 mg

Chili Tofu Noodles

SERVES 4 / PREP TIME: 5 MINUTES / COOK TIME: 15 MINUTES

Packs a punch!

---

1 cup green beans
2 cups rice noodles
1 tbsp coconut oil
6oz silken firm tofu, pressed & cubed
1/2 red chili, finely diced
1 garlic clove, minced
1 tsp fresh ginger, grated
1/2 lime, juiced

---

1. Steam the green beans for 10-12 minutes or according to package directions and drain.
2. Cook the noodles in a pot of boiling water (4 cups) for 10-15 minutes or according to package directions.
3. Meanwhile, heat a wok or skillet on a high heat and add coconut oil.
4. Now add the tofu, chili, garlic and ginger and sauté for 5-10 minutes.
5. Drain the noodles and add to the wok along with the green beans and lime juice.
6. Toss to coat.
7. Serve hot!

Per Serving: Calories 246
Protein 10 g
Carbohydrates 28g
Fat 12 g
Sodium 25 mg
Potassium 126 mg
Phosphorus 79 mg

Honey-Baked Spaghetti Squash

SERVES 4 / PREP TIME: 10 MINUTES / COOK TIME: 50 MINUTES

Often overlooked, spaghetti squash is delicious, fleshy and filling.

---

1 spaghetti squash
1 tbsp coconut oil
1 tbsp honey
1 red chili, de-seeded and sliced
2 cloves garlic, minced
2 cups baby spinach, washed

---

1. Pre-heat the oven to 375°F/190 °C/Gas Mark 5.
2. Once squash is prepared, place each side into a large oven dish (skin up).
3. Pour half a cup of water into the dish.
4. Bake for 45 minutes or until tender and remove the dish from the oven.
5. Meanwhile, mix the oil with the honey, chili and garlic and place to one side.
6. Turn the squash over and drizzle over the oil, garlic, honey and chili flakes.
7. Use a fork to shred the flesh from each half and serve on top of your choice of salad.

Per Serving: Calories 108
Protein 4 g
Carbohydrates 9 g
Fat 6 g
Sodium 254 mg
Potassium 85 mg
Phosphorus 34 mg

Vegetable Tagine

SERVES 2 / PREP TIME: 5 MINUTES / COOK TIME: 35 MINUTES

Who needs meat with these flavors!

---

2 tbsp coconut oil
1 onion, diced
1 turnip, peeled and diced
2 cloves of garlic
1 tsp ground cumin
1 tsp ground ginger
1 tsp ground cinnamon
1 tsp cayenne pepper
1 carrot, peeled and diced
1 red bell pepper, diced
1/2 can apricots, juices drained
3 cups water
2 tbsp lemon juice
2 tbsp cilantro, roughly chopped

---

1. Soak the vegetables in warm water prior to use.
2. In a large pot, heat the oil on a medium-high heat before sautéing the onion for 4-5 minutes until soft.
3. Add the turnip and cook for 10 minutes or until golden brown.
4. Add the garlic, cumin, ginger, cinnamon, and cayenne pepper, cooking for a further 3 minutes.
5. Add the carrots, red pepper, apricots and water to the pot and then bring to the boil.
6. Turn the heat down to a medium heat, cover and simmer for 20 minutes.
7. Add the lemon juice towards the end of cooking.
8. Garnish with the cilantro to serve.

Per Serving: Calories 208
Protein 2 g
Carbohydrates 22 g
Fat 15 g
Sodium 40 mg
Potassium 323 mg
Phosphorus 76 mg

Curried Cauliflower

SERVES 4 / PREP TIME: 5 MINUTES / COOK TIME: 20 MINUTES

Cauliflower is often used in Indian cuisine, due to its chunky texture and health benefits.

1 tbsp coconut oil
1 onion, diced
1 garlic clove, minced
1 tsp cumin
1 tsp turmeric
1 tsp garam masala
1/2 chili, diced
2 cups cauliflower, florets
1/2 cup water
1 tbsp fresh cilantro, chopped to garnish

1. Add the oil to a skillet on a medium heat.
2. Sauté the onion and garlic for 5 minutes until soft.
3. Add the cumin, turmeric and garam masala and stir to release the aromas.
4. Now add the chili to the pan along with the cauliflower.
5. Stir to coat.
6. Pour in the water and reduce the heat to a simmer for 15 minutes.
7. Garnish with cilantro to serve.

Per Serving: Calories 108
Protein 2 g
Carbohydrates 11 g
Fat 7 g
Sodium 35 mg
Potassium 328 mg
Phosphorus 39 mg

Roasted Mediterranean Veg

SERVES 6 / PREP TIME: 10 MINUTES / COOK TIME: 1 HOUR

Divine slow-roasted vegetables in olive oil and garlic.

---

2 onions, diced
2 zucchinis, diced
2 cups spaghetti squash, diced
1 cup eggplant, diced
2 medium carrots, diced
1 red bell pepper, diced
1 red chili pepper, diced
1 tbsp fresh basil
1 tbsp fresh oregano
1 tbsp fresh rosemary
1 tbsp fresh thyme
1 tbsp black pepper
2 tbsp extra virgin olive oil
2 garlic cloves, halved

---

1. Soak all vegetables in warm water prior to use.
2. Preheat the oven to 190°C/375°F/Gas Mark 5.
3. Add all of the vegetables, herbs and pepper to a shallow baking dish.
4. Drizzle with olive oil and scatter over the garlic cloves.
5. Roast in the oven for 45-60 minutes until tender.
6. Portion up and enjoy - you can add these to rice or pasta if you want a bigger meal.
7. Hint: Double up and save leftovers in an airtight container in the fridge for 2-3 days to snack on cold or heat through thoroughly to add to lunch.

Per Serving: Calories 101
Protein 2 g
Carbohydrates 13 g
Fat 4 g
Sodium 37 mg
Potassium 389 mg
Phosphorus 71 mg

Brie & Beet Frittata

SERVES 4 / PREP TIME: 5 MINUTES / COOK TIME: 25 MINUTES

Brie can be enjoyed occasionally if you can tolerate dairy.

---

8 egg whites
1 cup rice milk
1 tbsp coconut oil
1 cup canned beets, juices drained
1 tsp black pepper
1/2 cup brie, sliced

---

1. Preheat the broiler to a medium heat.
2. Whisk the eggs and rice milk in a mixing bowl.
3. In an oven proof (steel frying pan) add the oil and sauté the beets for 5 minutes. Sprinkle with black pepper.
4. Alternatively use a skillet and then transfer this into a tart dish afterwards.
5. Pour the egg mix into the pan.
6. Turn down to a low heat and leave for 7 minutes until the egg mixture becomes light and bubbly.
7. Scatter the sliced brie on the top of the mixture.
8. Finish the frittata in its pan/tart dish under the broiler for a further 5 -10 minutes or until crispy on the top and cooked through.
9. Slice and serve hot or allow to cool and serve chilled from the fridge!

Per Serving: Calories 187
Protein 12 g
Carbohydrates 5 g
Fat 5 g
Sodium 200 mg
Potassium 166 mg
Phosphorus 136 mg

Garlic & Arugula Pesto Pasta

SERVES 4 / PREP TIME: 5 MINUTES / COOK TIME: 20 MINUTES

So delicious!

---

2 cups fresh white penne pasta
1/2 cup fresh basil, washed
2 cups arugula, washed
1/4 cup extra virgin olive oil
2 garlic cloves, crushed
1 lemon, juiced

1 tsp black pepper

---

1. Bring a pan of water to the boil and add the pasta, cooking for 15-20 minutes or according to package directions.
2. Meanwhile, blend the rest of the ingredients in a food processor or a blender until smooth.
3. Drain the pasta and stir through the pesto over a very low heat until pesto is warmed through.
4. Serve with a sprinkle of black pepper to taste!

Per Serving: Calories 187
Protein 3 g
Carbohydrates 21 g
Fat 14 g
Sodium 18 mg
Potassium 51 mg
Phosphorus 50 mg

Chinese Tempeh Stir Fry

SERVES 2 / PREP TIME: 5 MINUTES / COOK TIME: 15 MINUTES

Quick and easy stir-fry dinner!

---

1 tbsp coconut oil
1 clove garlic, minced
1 tsp fresh ginger, minced
2oz tempeh, sliced
1/2 cup corn
1/2 cup green onions
1 cup white rice, cooked

---

1. Heat the oil in a skillet or wok on a high heat and add the garlic and ginger.
2. Sauté for 1 minute.
3. Now add the tempeh and cook for 5-6 minutes before adding the corn for a further 10 minutes.
4. Now add the green onions and serve over rice.

Per Serving: Calories 304
Protein 10 g
Carbohydrates 35 g
Fat 4 g
Sodium 91 mg
Potassium 121 mg
Phosphorus 22 mg

Veggie Pancakes

SERVES 2 / PREP TIME: 10 MINUTES / COOK TIME: 10 MINUTES

Savoury pancakes to enjoy for lunch or dinner.

1/2 red onion, finely diced
1/2 red bell pepper finely diced
3 tbsp extra virgin olive oil
1 tbsp mixed dried herbs
2 eggs
1/2 cup rice milk (unenriched)
1/2 cup water
1 tsp black pepper
1 cup white all-purpose flour

1. Soak the vegetables in warm water before cooking.
2. Preheat the broiler to a medium-high heat.
3. Add the vegetables to a baking tray; drizzle with 1 tbsp olive oil and sprinkle with the herbs.
4. Broil/grill for 10-15 minutes.
5. In a medium bowl whisk the eggs, milk, water, and pepper together until combined.
6. Add the flour to the mix and whisk into a smooth paste.
7. Melt the rest of the oil in a skillet over a medium heat.
8. Add 1/2 pancake mixture to form a round pancake shape.
9. Cook for 4-5 minutes until the bottom is light brown and easily comes away from the pan with the spatula.
10. Flip and add half the vegetables to the top before cooking for a further 4 minutes.
11. Fold and serve warm.
12. Serve and repeat with the rest of the ingredients.

Per Serving: Calories 325
Protein 7 g
Carbohydrates 15 g
Fat 25 g
Sodium 86 mg
Potassium 181 mg
Phosphorus 206 mg

Parsley Root Veg Stew

SERVES 4 / PREP TIME: 5 MINUTES / COOK TIME: 35-40 MINUTES

A vegetarian take on this classic dish.

---

2 tbsp olive oil
1 onion, diced
4 turnips, peeled and diced
2 cloves of garlic
1 tsp ground cumin
1 tsp ground ginger
1/2 tsp ground cinnamon
1 tsp cayenne pepper
2 carrots, peeled and diced
2 cups water
2 cups white rice + 4cups water
1/4 cup fresh parsley, chopped

---

1. In a large pot, heat the oil on a medium high heat before sautéing the onion for 4-5 minutes until soft.
2. Add the turnips and cook for 10 minutes or until golden brown.
3. Add the garlic, cumin, ginger, cinnamon, and cayenne pepper, cooking for a further 3 minutes.
4. Add the carrots and water to the pot and then bring to the boil.
5. Turn the heat down to a medium heat, cover and simmer for 20 minutes.
6. Meanwhile add the rice to a pot of water (4 cups) and bring to the boil.
7. Turn down to simmer for 15 minutes.
8. Drain and place the lid on for 5 minutes to steam.
9. Garnish the root vegetable stew with parsley to serve alongside the rice.

Per Serving: Calories 210
Protein 4 g
Carbohydrates 32 g
Fat 7 g
Sodium 67 mg
Potassium 181 mg
Phosphorus 105 mg

Mixed Pepper Paella

SERVES 2 / PREP TIME: 10 MINUTES / COOK TIME: 35-40 MINUTES

A delicious protein packed meal!

---

1 cup white rice
1 tbsp extra virgin olive oil
1/2 red bell pepper, chopped
1/2 yellow bell pepper, chopped
1/2 red onion, chopped
1/2 zucchini, chopped
1 tsp paprika
1 tsp oregano (dried)
1 tsp parsley (dried)
1 lemon

1 cup homemade chicken broth

---

1. Add the rice to a pot of cold water (2 cups) and cook for 15 minutes.
2. Drain the water, cover the pan and leave to one side.
3. Heat the oil in a skillet over a medium-high heat.
4. Add the bell pepper,s onion and zucchini, sautéing for 5 minutes.
5. To the pan, add the rice, herbs, spices and juice of the lemon along with the chicken broth.
6. Cover and turn heat right down and allow to simmer for 15-20 minutes.
7. Serve hot.

Per Serving: Calories 210
Protein 4 g
Carbohydrates 33 g
Fat 7 g
Sodium 20 mg
Potassium 33 mg
Phosphorus 156 mg

Cauliflower Rice & Runny Eggs

SERVES 4 / PREP TIME: 5 MINUTES / COOK TIME: 30 MINUTES

Yummy

---

2 cups cauliflower
1 tbsp extra virgin olive oil
1 tbsp curry powder
1 tsp black pepper
4 eggs

1 tbsp fresh chives, chopped

---

1. Preheat the oven to 375°f/190°c/Gas Mark 5.
2. Soak the cauliflower in warm water in advance if possible.
3. Grate or chop into rice-size pieces.
4. Bring the cauliflower to the boil in a pot of water (to cover cauliflower) and then turn down to simmer for 7 minutes.
5. Drain completely.
6. Place on a baking tray and sprinkle over curry powder and black pepper - toss to coat.
7. Bake in the oven for 20 minutes, stirring occasionally.
8. Meanwhile, boil a separate pan of water and add the eggs for 7 minutes.
9. Run under the cold tap, crack and peel the eggs before cutting in half.
10. Top the cauliflower with eggs and chopped chives.
11. Serve hot!

Per Serving: Calories 120
Protein 7 g
Carbohydrates 4 g
Fat 8 g
Sodium 175 mg
Potassium 188 mg
Phosphorus 134 mg

Minted Zucchini Noodles

SERVES 2 / PREP TIME: 5 MINUTES / COOK TIME: 10 MINUTES

Fresh and light noodles with an lemony arugula topping.

1/2 cup fresh mint, chopped
1 tsp black pepper
1/4 red chili, de-seeded and chopped
2 tbsp extra virgin olive oil1
4 zucchinis, peeled and sliced
vertically to make noodles (use a spiral-
izer)
1/2 cup arugula
1/2 lemon, juiced

---

1. Whisk the mint, pepper, chili and olive oil to make a dressing.
2. Meanwhile, heat a pan of water on a high heat and bring to the boil.
3. Add the zucchini noodles and turn the heat down to simmer for 3-4 minutes.
4. Remove from the heat and place in a bowl of cold water immediately.
5. Toss the noodles in the dressing.
6. Mix the arugula with the lemon juice to serve on the top.
7. Enjoy!

Per Serving: Calories 148
Protein 2 g
Carbohydrates 4 g
Fat 13 g
Sodium 7 mg
Potassium 422 mg
Phosphorus 256 mg

Curried Eggplant

SERVES 2 / PREP TIME: 10 MINUTES / COOK TIME: 40 MINUTES

Aromatic vegan dish.

---

1 tbsp coconut oil
1/2 red onion, finely diced
1 garlic clove, minced
1 cup eggplant, peeled and cubed
1 tbsp curry powder
1 tsp garam masala
1 tsp cumin
1/2 cup water
1 cup white rice, cooked
2 tbsp fresh cilantro, chopped

---

1. Soak vegetables in warm water prior to cooking.
2. Preheat the oven to 350°f/170°c/Gas Mark 4.
3. Add the coconut oil to a pan or skillet over a medium heat.
4. Add the onions and garlic to the pan and sauté for 5-6 minutes.
5. Now add the eggplant cubes and sauté for 5 minutes.
6. Sprinkle in the curry powder and spices and stir to coat.
7. Add 1/2 cup water, cover and simmer for 30 minutes or until eggplant is soft.
8. Keep an eye on water levels so as not to let it stick or burn.
9. Serve over rice and scatter with fresh cilantro.

Per Serving: Calories 221
Protein 4 g
Carbohydrates 31 g
Fat 8 g
Sodium 193 mg
Potassium 243 mg
Phosphorus 108 mg

Chili Tempeh & Scallions

SERVES 2 / PREP TIME: 10 MINUTES / COOK TIME: 15 MINUTES

Chunky tempeh with a kick.

---

1 tsp coconut oil
1 tsp soy sauce (reduced sodium)
1 lime, juiced
1 tbsp ginger, grated
1/2 red chili, de-seeded and chopped
2oz tempeh, cubed
1/2 cup scallions, chopped

---

1. Mix the oil, soy sauce, chili flakes, lime juice and ginger together.
2. Marinate the tempeh in this for as long as possible.
3. Preheat the broiler to a medium heat.
4. Add tempeh to a lined baking tray and broil for 10-15 minutes or until hot through.
5. Remove and sprinkle with scallions to serve.

Per Serving: Calories 221
Protein 6 g
Carbohydrates 8 g
Fat 10 g
Sodium 466 mg
Potassium 189 mg
Phosphorus 99 mg

SEAFOOD

Shrimp Paella

SERVES 2 / PREP TIME: 5 MINUTES / COOK TIME: 10 MINUTES

Tasty seafood dish.

---

1 tbsp olive oil
1 red onion, chopped
1 garlic clove, chopped
6 oz frozen cooked shrimp
1 tsp paprika
1 chili pepper, de-seeded and sliced
1 tbsp oregano
1 cup cooked white rice

---

1. Heat the olive oil in a large pan on a medium-high heat.
2. Add the onion and garlic and sauté for 2-3 minutes until soft.
3. Now add the shrimp and sauté for a further 5 minutes or until hot through.
4. Now add the herbs,spices, chili and rice with 1/2 cup boiling water.
5. Stir until everything is warm and the water has been absorbed.
6. Plate up and serve.

Per Serving: Calories 221
Protein 17 g
Carbohydrates 31 g
Fat 8 g
Sodium 235 mg
Potassium 176 mg
Phosphorus 189 mg

Salmon & Pesto Salad

SERVES 2 / PREP TIME: 5 MINUTES / COOK TIME: 15 MINUTES

Add a little twist to your normal salmon dish.

For the pesto:

1/2 cup fresh basil
1/2 cup fresh arugula
1 tsp black pepper
1/4 cup extra virgin olive oil
1 garlic clove, minced

For the salmon:

1 tbsp coconut oil
4oz salmon fillet, skinless

For the salad:
1/2 cup iceberg lettuce, washed

2 radishes, sliced
1/2 lemon, juiced
1 tsp black pepper

1. Prepare the pesto by blending all the ingredients for the pesto in a food processor or by grinding with a pestle and mortar.
2. Place to one side.
3. Add a skillet to the stove on a medium-high heat and melt the coconut oil.
4. Add the salmon to the pan.
5. Cook for 7-8 minutes and turn over.
6. Cook for a further 3-4 minutes or until cooked through.
7. Remove fillets from the skillet and allow to rest.
8. Mix the lettuce and the radishes and squeeze over juice of 1/2 lemon.
9. Flake the salmon with a fork and mix through the salad.
10. Toss to coat and sprinkle with a little black pepper to serve.

Per Serving: Calories 221
Protein 13 g
Carbohydrates 1 g
Fat 34 g
Sodium 80 mg
Potassium 119 mg
Phosphorus 158 mg

Baked Fennel & Garlic Sea Bass

SERVES 2 / PREP TIME: 5 MINUTES / COOK TIME: 15 MINUTES

Juicy and flavorsome,

---

1 tsp black pepper
2x 3oz sea bass fillets
1/2 fennel bulb, sliced
2 garlic cloves
1 lemon

---

1. Preheat the oven to 375°f/190°c/Gas Mark 5.
2. Sprinkle black pepper over the sea bass.
3. Slice the fennel bulb and garlic cloves.
4. Add 1 sea bass fillet and half the fennel and garlic to one sheet of baking paper or tin foil.
5. Squeeze in 1/2 lemon juices.
6. Repeat for the other fillet.
7. Fold and add to the oven for 12-15 minutes or until fish is thoroughly cooked through.
8. Serve with your choice of rice or salad.

Per Serving: Calories 221
Protein 14 g
Carbohydrates 3 g
Fat 2 g
Sodium 119 mg
Potassium 398 mg
Phosphorus 149 mg

Lemon, Garlic & Cilantro Tuna With Rice

SERVES 2 / PREP TIME: 5 MINUTES / COOK TIME: NA

Prepare in advance for a go-to lunch!

---

1 tbsp extra virgin olive oil
1 tsp black pepper
2 tbsp fresh cilantro, chopped
1/4 red onion, finely diced
1 lemon, juiced
4oz canned tuna in water
1 cup rice, cooked
1/2 cup arugula, washed

---

1. Mix the olive oil, pepper, cilantro, red onion in a and lemon juice bowl.
2. Stir in the tuna , cover and leave in the fridge for as long as possible (if you can) or serve immediately.
3. When ready to eat, serve up with the cooked rice and arugula!

Per Serving: Calories 221
Protein 11 g
Carbohydrates 26 g
Fat 7 g
Sodium 143 mg
Potassium 197 mg
Phosphorus 182 mg

Cod & Green Bean Risotto

SERVES 2 / PREP TIME: 4 MINUTES / COOK TIME: 40 MINUTES

Soft and succulent lemon-infused fish risotto.

---

1 tbsp extra virgin olive oil
1 white onion, finely diced
1 cup white rice
1 cup low sodium chicken broth (see soups and stocks chapter)
1 cup boiling water
1/2 cup of green beans
4oz cod fillet
Pinch of black pepper
2 lemon wedges
1/2 cup arugula

---

1. Heat the oil in a large pan on a medium heat.
2. Sauté the chopped onion for 5 minutes until soft before adding in the rice and stirring for 1-2 minutes.
3. Combine the broth with boiling water in a measuring jug.
4. Add half of the liquid to the pan and stir slowly.
5. Slowly add the rest of the liquid whilst continuously stirring for up to 20-30 minutes.
6. Stir in the green beans to the risotto.
7. Place the fish on top of the rice, cover and steam for 10 minutes.
8. Ensure the water does not dry out and keep topping up until the rice is cooked thoroughly.
9. Use your fork to break up the fish fillets and stir into the rice.
10. Sprinkle with freshly ground pepper to serve and a squeeze of fresh lemon.
11. Garnish with the lemon wedges and serve with the arugula.

Per Serving: Calories 221
Protein 12 g
Carbohydrates 29 g
Fat 8 g
Sodium   398 mg
Potassium 347 mg
Phosphorus 241 mg

Mixed Pepper Stuffed River Trout

SERVES 4 / PREP TIME: 5 MINUTES / COOK TIME: 20 MINUTES

This tastes scrumptious and fresh!

---

1 tsp extra virgin olive oil
1/4 red pepper, diced
1/4 yellow pepper, diced
1/4 green pepper, diced
1 tsp thyme
1 tsp oregano
1 tsp black pepper
1 cup baby spinach leaves, washed
1 lime, juiced
1 whole river trout (8oz), skinned and

gutted by your fishmonger

---

1. Preheat the broiler /grill on a high heat.
2. Lightly oil a baking tray.
3. Mix all of the ingredients apart from the trout and lime.
4. Slice the trout lengthways (there should be an opening here from where it was gutted) and stuff the mixed ingredients inside.
5. Squeeze the lime juice over the fish and then place the lime wedges on the tray.
6. Place under the broiler on the baking tray and broil for 15-20 minutes or until fish is thoroughly cooked through and flakes easily.
7. Enjoy alone or with a side helping of rice or salad.

Per Serving: Calories 290
Protein 15 g
Carbohydrates 0 g
Fat 7 g
Sodium   43 mg
Potassium 315 mg
Phosphorus 189 mg

Mahi Mahi & Salsa

SERVES 2 / PREP TIME: 10 MINUTES / COOK TIME: 10 MINUTES

A wonderfully meaty fish with a Mexican style salsa.

---

1 tbsp coconut oil
2x 3oz fresh mahi mahi fillets, skinless
1/4 red bell pepper, finely diced
1/4 red onion, finely diced
2 tbsp fresh cilantro
2 tbsp olive oil
1 tsp black pepper
1 lime, juiced
1/4 cup arugula

---

1. Heat the coconut oil in a pan on a medium-high heat.
2. Add the mahi mahi fillets and cook for 5 minutes.
3. Turn over and cook for a further 5 minutes.
4. Meanwhile, prepare the salsa by mixing the bell pepper, onion, cilantro, pepper and oil in a separate bowl.
5. Squeeze in the lime juice.
6. Wash the arugula.
7. Serve each mahi mahi fillet with a side helping of salsa and arugula.

Per Serving: Calories 207
Protein 16 g
Carbohydrates 4 g
Fat 14 g
Sodium 80 mg
Potassium 465 mg
Phosphorus 90 mg

Basil & Lemon Swordfish Kebabs

SERVES 2 / PREP TIME: 30 MINUTES / COOK TIME: 10 MINUTES

A great alternative to chicken and lamb - try cooking on the BBQ on a hot day!

4oz swordfish fillet, skinless
1 lemon
2 tbsp fresh basil, chopped
1 tsp curry powder
1/2 lemon juiced
1 tbsp extra virgin olive oil
1/2 green bell pepper (8 pieces)
1/2 red onion (8 pieces)

---

1. Soak the vegetables in warm water before cooking.
2. Cut the swordfish into 8 bite-size pieces.
3. Whisk the basil, onion, curry powder, lemon juice and oil to form a brushing oil for your swordfish.
4. Skewer 1 piece of pepper, then 1 piece of red onion then 1 piece of swordfish.
5. Repeat until you have 4 slices of swordfish on each skewer.
6. Use a basting brush to coat the swordfish and vegetables with the cooking oil.
7. Cover and marinate in the refrigerator for at least 30 minutes.
8. Preheat the broiler to a medium heat when ready to cook.
9. Place kebabs on an oven dish under the broiler for 8 minutes.
10. Turn skewers to brown each side.
11. Serve hot.

Per Serving: Calories 207
Protein 16 g
Carbohydrates 10 g
Fat 14 g
Sodium   318 mg
Potassium 404 mg
Phosphorus 215 mg

Haddock & Buttered Leeks

SERVES 2 / PREP TIME: 5 MINUTES / COOK TIME: 15 MINUTES

A simple yet divine recipe .

2x 3oz haddock fillets
Pinch of black pepper
1/2 lemon, juiced
1 tbsp unsalted butter
1 leek, sliced widthways
2 tsp parsley, chopped

---

1. Preheat the oven to 375°f/190°c/Gas Mark 5.
2. Add the haddock fillets to baking or parchment paper and sprinkle with the black pepper.
3. Squeeze over the lemon juice and wrap into a parcel.
4. Bake the parcel on a baking tray for 10-15 minutes or until fish is thoroughly cooked through.
5. Meanwhile, heat the butter over a medium-low heat in a small pan.
6. Add the leeks and parsley and sauté for 5-7 minutes until soft.
7. Serve the haddock fillets on a bed of buttered leeks and enjoy!

Per Serving: Calories 124
Protein 15 g
Carbohydrates 0 g
Fat 7 g
Sodium 161 mg
Potassium 251 mg
Phosphorus 220 mg

Thai Spiced Halibut

SERVES 2   PREP TIME: 5 MINUTES   COOK TIME: 20 MINUTES

Bring a taste of Thailand to your dinner table.

4oz halibut fillet
Pinch of black pepper
2 garlic cloves, pressed
2 tbsp coconut oil
1 lime, halved
1/2 red chilli, diced
2 green onions, sliced
1 lime leaf
1 tbsp fresh basil
Cup of white rice

---

1. Preheat oven to 400°f/190°c/Gas Mark 5.
2. Add half of the ingredients into baking paper and fold into a parcel.
3. Repeat for your second parcel.
4. Add to the oven for 15-20 minutes or until fish is thoroughly cooked through.
5. Serve with cooked rice.

Per Serving: Calories 311
Protein 16 g
Carbohydrates 17 g
Fat 15 g
Sodium   31 mg
Potassium 418 mg
Phosphorus 261 mg

Homemade Tuna Nicoise

SERVES 2 / PREP TIME: 5 MINUTES / COOK TIME: 10 MINUTES

A wholesome salad, good enough for any main meal.

---

4 iceberg lettuce leaves
1/4 cucumber, thinly sliced
1/4 red onion, thinly sliced
4oz canned tuna in water, drained
1 tbsp olive oil
1 lemon, juiced
1 tsp fresh cilantro, chopped
1 tbsp capers
1 egg
1/2 cup green beans
1 tsp black pepper

---

1. Prepare the salad by washing and slicing the lettuce, cucumber and onion.
2. Add to a salad bowl.
3. Mix 1 tbsp oil with the lemon juice, cilantro and capers for a salad dressing.
4. Place to one side.
5. Boil a pan of water on a high heat then lower to simmer and add the egg for 6 minutes. (Steam the green beans over the same pan in a steamer/colander for the 6 minutes).
6. Remove the egg and rinse under cold water.
7. Peel before slicing in half.
8. Mix the tuna, salad and dressing together in a salad bowl.
9. Toss to coat.
10. Top with the egg and serve with a sprinkle of black pepper.

Per Serving: Calories 199
Protein 19 g
Carbohydrates 7 g
Fat 8 g
Sodium 466 mg
Potassium 251 mg
Phosphorus 211 mg

Monk Fish Curry

SERVES 2 / PREP TIME: 5 MINUTES / COOK TIME: 20 MINUTES

A perfect fish for curries.

4oz monk fish fillet
2 tsp fresh basil, chopped
1 garlic clove
1 tsp ginger, grated
1/2 red chili, finely sliced
1/2 stick lemon-grass, finely sliced
1 tbsp coconut oil
2 tbsp shallots, chopped
1 cup water
1 cup rice noodles, cooked

3 green onions, finely chopped

---

1. Slice the Monkfish into bite-size pieces.
2. Using a pestle and mortar or food processor, crush the basil, garlic, ginger, chili and lemon-grass to form a paste.
3. Heat the oil in a large wok or pan over a medium-high heat and add the shallots.
4. Now add the water to the pan and bring to the boil.
5. Add the Monkfish, lower the heat and cover to simmer for 10 minutes or until cooked through.
6. Enjoy with rice noodles and scatter with green onions to serve.

Per Serving: Calories 249
Protein 12 g
Carbohydrates 30 g
Fat 10 g
Sodium   32 mg
Potassium 398 mg
Phosphorus 190 mg

Chili & Lime Crab Tortillas

SERVES 4 / PREP TIME: 5 MINUTES / COOK TIME: 15 MINUTES

Too tempting!

---

8 oz crab meat
2 scallions, washed and sliced
1/4 green chili, finely sliced
1 lime
1 tsp coconut oil
4 tortillas
1 cup arugula, washed
1/2 cucumber, peeled & sliced

---

1. Mix the crab meat, scallions, chili and lime juice in a bowl.
2. Heat the coconut oil in a wok or skillet over a medium heat.
3. Add the crab meat mix to the skillet and cook for 10 minutes, stirring occasionally.
4. Add the tortillas to the microwave or grill for 1 minute.
5. Layer the centre of each tortilla with arugula and cucumber before topping with a quarter of the crab mixture.
6. Roll into a wrap your style!
7. Repeat for the rest of the mixture and serve.

Per Serving: Calories 198
Protein 15 g
Carbohydrates 20 g
Fat 6 g
Sodium 169 mg
Potassium 195 mg
Phosphorus 197 mg

Honey Salmon & Spaghetti Squash

SERVES 8 / PREP TIME: 10 MINUTES / COOK TIME: 45 MINUTES

This dish is magnificent!

---

1 spaghetti squash (approx. 4 cups)
16oz skinless salmon fillets
1 tbsp extra virgin olive oil
1 tbsp honey
1/2 red chili, finely diced
1 garlic clove, minced
1 tsp coconut oil
2 cups green beans, cooked
A pinch of black pepper

---

1. Pre-heat the oven to 375°F/190 °C/Gas Mark 5.
2. Cut squash in half lengthways.
3. Place each side into a large oven dish (skin up).
4. Pour half a cup of water into the dish.
5. Bake for 45 minutes or until tender .
6. Meanwhile, mix the olive oil with the honey, chili and garlic and place to one side.
7. Coat the salmon fillets with the marinade (you could do this the night before for extra flavor).
8. Heat the coconut oil in a large pan or skillet over a medium-high heat and add the salmon fillets.
9. Cook for 6-8 minutes each side or until completely cooked through.
10. When squash is tender through to the centre, remove from the oven and place to one side to cool.
11. Use a fork to shred the flesh from each half of the squash.
12. Serve the salmon on top of a bed of flaked spaghetti squash with a side of green beans.

Per Serving: Calories 144
Protein 11 g
Carbohydrates 6 g
Fat 8 g
Sodium 128 mg
Potassium 278 mg
Phosphorus 166 mg

Scallops With Pineapple & Chili

SERVES 2 / PREP TIME: 5 MINUTES / COOK TIME: 10 MINUTES

A special treat.

1/4 cup canned pineapple, drained
1/4 red onion, finely diced
1 red chilli, diced
1/2 garlic clove, minced
1 tbsp coconut oil
5oz scallops
1/2 lime, juiced
Pinch of black pepper

---

1. Finely dice the pineapple pieces and mix with the red onion, chili and garlic.
2. Heat the oil in a pan or skillet over a medium-high heat.
3. Add the pineapple mix to the pan for 5 minutes, stirring so the onion doesn't brown.
4. Make a space in the centre of the pan for the scallops.
5. Add the scallops to the pan and cook for 2-3 minutes each side.
6. Gently shake the pan a little so that the pineapple juices cook with the scallops.
7. Squeeze over the lime juice for the last minute in the pan.
8. Sprinkle with black pepper and enjoy!

Per Serving: Calories 141
Protein 11 g
Carbohydrates 10 g
Fat 7 g
Sodium 278 mg
Potassium 254 mg
Phosphorus 258 mg

Sweet & Sour Shrimp

SERVES 2 / PREP TIME: 30 MINUTES / COOK TIME: 15 MINUTES

This dish is so easy to cook and tastes sublime.

---

4 tsp fresh cilantro
1 onion, finely diced
1/2 lemon, juiced
1 tbsp coconut oil
1 garlic clove, minced

1/4 cup canned pineapple, cubed and drained
4 oz raw shrimp
1 cup rice noodles

---

1. Whisk cilantro, onion, lemon juice, oil and garlic in a separate bowl.
2. Add the pineapple chunks to the marinade.
3. Pour the marinade over the shrimps.
4. Cover and marinate in the refrigerator for at least 30 minutes.
5. Add the noodles to a pan of boiling water (2 cups) for 10-15 minutes or according to package directions.
6. Heat a wok or skillet over a medium-high heat.
7. Add the shrimp with the marinade, and sauté for 10-15 minutes or until thoroughly cooked through (shrimp should be pink and opaque).
8. Drain noodles and add to the wok.
9. Toss and enjoy.

Per Serving: Calories 228
Protein 16 g
Carbohydrates 31 g
Fat 7 g
Sodium 247 mg
Potassium 240 mg
Phosphorus 112 mg

Herby Swordfish Steaks

SERVES 2 / PREP TIME: 35 MINUTES / COOK TIME: 40 MINUTES

If you can't get hold of swordfish, try this with tuna, shark or monk fish.

---

1 tbsp basil, fresh or dried
1 tbsp thyme, fresh or dried
Pinch of black pepper
1 garlic clove, minced
1/2 lemon
2 tbsp extra virgin olive oil
4oz swordfish steak, skinless
1 cup watercress, washed

---

1. In a bowl, mix the herbs, pepper, garlic, lemon juice and olive oil.
2. Marinate the swordfish steak for at least 30 minutes.
3. Preheat oven to 325°f/150°c/Gas Mark 3.
4. Bake the fish in parchment paper for 30-40 minutes, until well cooked.
5. Slice the swordfish and serve on a bed of watercress.

Per Serving: Calories 210
Protein 15 g
Carbohydrates 1 g
Fat 15 g
Sodium 138 mg
Potassium 280 mg
Phosphorus 214 mg

Asian Fish Soup

SERVES 4 / PREP TIME: 5 MINUTES / COOK TIME: 25 MINUTES

A taste of the Far-East!

---

1 tsp black pepper
2 cups water
1 tsp coconut oil
1 tsp five-spice powder
1 tbsp olive oil
1 tbsp ginger, minced
1 cup rice noodles
1 green onion, thinly sliced
1/4 cup canned corn
8oz cod/haddock fillet, skinless and de-boned
2 tsp cilantro, finely chopped

---

1. In a bowl, combine black pepper, 1 1/2 cups of water, coconut oil and five-spice.
2. In a large saucepan, heat the olive oil on a medium heat and sauté the ginger for 2 minutes.
3. Add the rest of the water to the saucepan and heat through for 5 minutes.
4. Add the noodles to the pan and stir, bringing to a simmer over a high heat.
5. Add the green onion, corn and the fish and cook for 10-15 minutes until fish is tender and cooked through.
6. Garnish with the cilantro to serve.

Per Serving: Calories 181
Protein 12 g
Carbohydrates 16 g
Fat 8 g
Sodium 132 mg
Potassium 336 mg
Phosphorus 149 mg

Garlic Shrimp Tagliatelle

SERVES 4 / PREP TIME: 5 MINUTES / COOK TIME: 20 MINUTES

Another winner.

6oz shrimp, fresh or frozen
2 cups tagliatelle, dried
2 tbsp olive oil
1 garlic clove, minced
1/4 cup scallions, chopped
1 lemon, juiced
1 cup arugula

---

1. If the shrimp is frozen, allow to thoroughly defrost before cooking.
2. Heat a pan of water (5 cups) over a medium-high heat.
3. Once boiling, add the tagliatelle and lower heat to a simmer.
4. Cook according to package directions.
5. Meanwhile, heat 1 tbsp oil in a skillet over a medium heat.
6. Add the garlic and scallions and sauté for 1-2 minutes.
7. Now add the shrimp and cook thoroughly according to package directions.
8. Squeeze 1/4 lemon juice into the pan and shake gently for 1-2 minutes.
9. Drain the pasta and pour the shrimp, scallions and all the lovely juices over the top.
10. Toss to coat
11. Drizzle the rest of the olive oil and lemon juice over the linguine to serve with a helping of arugula on top.

Per Serving: Calories 263
Protein 17 g
Carbohydrates 7 g
Fat 7 g
Sodium 17 mg
Potassium 112 mg
Phosphorus 109 mg

Haddock & Parsley Fish Cakes

SERVES 2 / PREP TIME: 5 MINUTES / COOK TIME: 40 MINUTES

Great for the kidneys!

---

2 turnips, peeled and cubed
4oz haddock fillets, skinless
2 cups rice milk (unenriched)
1 tsp black pepper
2 tbsp extra virgin olive oil
2 tbsp fresh or dried parsley
1/2 cup fresh spinach
1 tsp black pepper
1/2 lemon

---

1. Soak all your vegetables in warm water prior to use.
2. Pre-heat the oven to 375°F/190 °C/Gas Mark 5.
3. Boil a pan of water on a high heat and add the turnips.
4. Allow to boil for 20-25 minutes or until very soft.
5. Meanwhile, poach the haddock fillets in a pan of rice milk by bringing to the boil and then turning down to simmer for 20 minutes or until cooked through.
6. Drain haddock and flake with a fork in a mixing bowl.
7. Drain turnips and use a potato masher to mash.
8. Combine with the flaked haddock.
9. Add black pepper, 1 tbsp olive oil, herbs and spinach.
10. Shape mixture into 2 fish cakes (patties) with your palms.
11. Now grab a skillet and heat the rest of the oil over a medium-high heat.
12. Cook the fish cakes for 7-8 minutes and turn over.
13. Cook for a further 3-4 minutes until golden brown on each side.
14. Remove and serve with your choice of vegetables, a squeeze of lemon and a pinch of black pepper.

Per Serving: Calories 322
Protein 12 g
Carbohydrates 35 g
Fat 16 g
Sodium 295 mg
Potassium 472 mg
Phosphorus 218 mg

Cod En Papillote

SERVES 4 / PREP TIME: 5 MINUTES / COOK TIME: 20 MINUTES

Mediterranean flavors in a juicy parcel!

8oz cod fillets, skinless & de-boned
1 lemon, halved
1 tbsp olive oil
1 garlic clove, minced
1/4 red onion, sliced
1 cup baby spinach leaves
1/4 zucchini, peeled and diced
1/4 red bell pepper, diced
1 cup white rice, cooked

---

1. Preheat oven to 400°f/200°c/Gas Mark 6.
2. Add all of the ingredients to a large sheet of baking paper or baking foil.
3. Squeeze the lemon juice over the fish before popping in the wedges.
4. Place in the oven for 15-20 minutes or until cooked through.
5. Divide into portions and serve hot!

Per Serving: Calories 148
Protein 14 g
Carbohydrates 15 g
Fat 4 g
Sodium 96 mg
Potassium 256 mg
Phosphorus 116 mg

Haddock & Spinach Crumble

SERVES 4 / PREP TIME: 35 MINUTES / COOK TIME: 1 HOUR

A lean fish pie.

---

2 cups rice milk (un-enriched)
8oz haddock fillets, skinless & boneless
1 tsp black pepper
1 tsp parsley
1/4 cup white breadcrumbs
1 cup cooked green beans, finely sliced

2 cups baby spinach

---

1. Preheat the oven to 400°f/200°c/Gas Mark 6.
2. Add the milk into a pan over a medium-high heat and bring to a simmer.
3. Add the haddock fillets, black pepper and parsley to the pan and lower the heat slightly.
4. Allow to simmer for 20-25 minutes or until cooked through.
5. Meanwhile, add the breadcrumbs, sliced green beans and spinach to a food processor and blitz together for 30 seconds for a grainy texture.
6. Use a fork to flake the haddock fillets once cooked and return to the milk.
7. Into a deep oven dish, add the haddock and milk.
8. Top with the crispy spinach mixture and bake in the oven for 25-30 minutes or until golden.

Per Serving: Calories 151
Protein 12 g
Carbohydrates 22 g
Fat 1 g
Sodium 183 mg
Potassium 524 mg
Phosphorus 173 mg

Seafood Sticks & Dill Salad

SERVES 4 / PREP TIME: 5 MINUTES / COOK TIME: 10 MINUTES

A lovely meal cooked under the grill or on the BBQ.

8oz scallops, cut into bite-size pieces
4 kebab sticks (metal)
1/2 lemon, juiced
1/2 cucumber
1 tsp dill
1 tbsp olive oil

---

1. Preheat the broiler or BBQ to a high heat.
2. Skewer the kebab sticks with the scallop pieces.
3. Squeeze the lemon juice over the top of the kebabs.
4. Broil on a lined baking tray for 4-5 minutes or until scallops are thoroughly cooked through.
5. Peel and slice the cucumber length ways.
6. Mix with the dill and olive oil
7. Serve the cucumber salad on the side of the kebabs.

Per Serving: Calories 146
Protein 17 g
Carbohydrates 5 g
Fat 7 g
Sodium 226 mg
Potassium 139 mg
Phosphorus 200 mg

SOUPS & STOCKS

Low-Sodium Chicken Broth

SERVES 2 / PREP TIME: 10 MINUTES / COOK TIME: 4 HOURS

This homemade chicken stock is far healthier than shop bought and can be used in some of the recipes featured in this cookbook. It's delicious too.

1 whole roasting chicken {around 4-5lbs}, skinless
3 carrots, soaked in warm water
2 medium onions
4 garlic cloves, crushed
2 bay leaves
3 stalks of celery, soaked in warm water

1 tbsp each dried rosemary, thyme, pepper, turmeric
1 tbsp white wine vinegar
11-12 cups water

1. Place chicken in a large saucepan or soup pan.
2. Peel and chop your vegetables into large chunks - add to the pan.
3. Add the rest of the ingredients to the pan.
4. Fill your pan with water so that the chicken and vegetables are completely covered.
5. Turn up to a high heat and bring to boiling point before reducing the heat and allowing the stock to simmer for 3-4 hours.
6. Top up with water if the ingredients become uncovered.
7. Turn the heat off and carefully remove the chicken, placing to one side.
8. Strain the liquid through a sieve into a separate bowl.
9. Leave the stock and chicken to cool.
10. Once cool, tear or cut the meat from the bones.
11. Add the broth to a sealed container and keep in the fridge (3 days) or freezer (3 months).
12. You can use the chicken meat for another dish.

Per cup : Calories 38
Protein 5 g
Carbohydrates 3 g
Fat 1 g
Sodium 72 mg
Potassium 197 mg
Phosphorus 72 mg

Paprika Pork Soup

SERVES 2 / PREP TIME: 5 MINUTES / COOK TIME: 35 MINUTES

Fragrant and wholesome soup.

---

1 tbsp extra-virgin olive oil
1 onion, chopped
2 garlic cloves, minced
4oz pork loin, sliced
1 tbsp paprika
3 cups water
1 cup baby spinach
1 tsp black pepper

---

1. In a large pot, add the oil, chopped onion and minced garlic.
2. Sauté for 5 minutes on a low heat.
3. Rub the pork slices with paprika.
4. Add the pork slices to the onions and cook for 7-8 minutes or until browned.
5. Add the water to the pan and bring to a boil on a high heat.
6. Stir in the spinach, reduce heat and simmer for a further 20 minutes or until pork is thoroughly cooked through.
7. Season with pepper to serve.

Per Serving: Calories 165
Protein 13 g
Carbohydrates 10 g
Fat 9 g
Sodium 269 mg
Potassium 486 mg
Phosphorus 158 mg

Spaghetti Squash & Yellow Bell-Pepper Soup

SERVES 4 / PREP TIME: 10 MINUTES / COOK TIME: 35 MINUTES

Another winter-warmer!

---

1 tbsp coconut oil
1 onion, quartered and sliced
2 large garlic cloves, chopped
1 tsp curry powder
4 cups water
1 spaghetti squash (approx. 4 cups),
peeled and cubed
2 yellow bell peppers, diced

1 sprig of thyme/1 tbsp dried thyme

---

1. Heat the oil in a large pan over a medium-high heat before sweating the onions and garlic for 3-4 minutes.
2. Sprinkle over the curry powder.
3. Add the water to the pan and bring to a boil over a high heat before adding the squash, peppers and thyme.
4. Turn down the heat, cover and allow to simmer for 25-30 minutes.
5. Continue to simmer until squash is soft if needed.
6. Allow to cool before blitzing in a blender/food processor until smooth.
7. Serve!

Per Serving: Calories 103
Protein 2 g
Carbohydrates 17 g
Fat 4 g
Sodium 32 mg
Potassium 365 mg
Phosphorus 50 mg

Red Pepper & Brie Soup

SERVES 4 / PREP TIME: 10 MINUTES / COOK TIME: 35 MINUTES

The sweetness of the peppers tastes delicious with the creamy brie.

---

2 tbsp of extra virgin olive oil
1 red onion, chopped
4 red bell peppers, chopped
2 garlic cloves, chopped
1 tsp cumin
1 tsp paprika
4 cups water
1/4 cup brie, crumbled

---

1. Heat the oil in a pot over a medium heat.
2. Sweat the onions and peppers for 5 minutes.
3. Add the garlic cloves, cumin and paprika and sauté for 3-4 minutes.
4. Add the water to the pot and allow to boil before turning heat down to simmer for 30 minutes.
5. Remove from the heat and allow to cool slightly.
6. Put the mixture in a food processor and blend until smooth.
7. Pour into serving bowls and add the crumbled brie to the top with a little black pepper.
8. Enjoy!

Per Serving: Calories 152
Protein 3 g
Carbohydrates 8 g
Fat 11 g
Sodium 66 mg
Potassium 270 mg
Phosphorus 207 mg

Turkey & Lemon-Grass Soup

SERVES 4 / PREP TIME: 5 MINUTES / COOK TIME: 40 MINUTES

Don't miss out on this chunky Asian-infused soup.

1/2 stick lemon-grass, finely sliced
1 tbsp cilantro
1 green chili, finely chopped
1 tbsp coconut oil
1/4 cup fresh basil leaves
1 white onion, chopped
1 garlic clove, minced
1 thumb size piece of minced ginger
4oz skinless turkey breasts, sliced
4 cups water
1 cup canned water chestnuts, drained
2 scallions, chopped
1 fresh lime

---

1. Crush the lemon-grass, cilantro, chili, 1/2 tbsp coconut oil and basil leaves in a blender or pestle and mortar to form a paste.
2. Heat a large pan/wok with 1/2 tbsp coconut oil on a high heat.
3. Sauté the onions, garlic and ginger until soft.
4. Add the turkey and brown each side for 4-5 minutes.
5. Add the water and stir.
6. Next add the water chestnuts, turn down the heat slightly and allow to simmer for 25-30 minutes or until turkey is thoroughly cooked through.
7. Serve hot with the scallions sprinkled over the top and a squeeze of lime juice.

Per Serving: Calories 123
Protein 10 g
Carbohydrates 12 g
Fat 3 g
Sodium 501 mg
Potassium 151 mg
Phosphorus 110 mg

Leek & Cauliflower Soup

SERVES 4 / PREP TIME: 10 MINUTES / COOK TIME: 40 MINUTES

Vegetarian and delicious.

---

2 tbsp coconut oil
2 leeks, finely sliced
4 cloves garlic, minced
2 cups cauliflower, chopped
1/2 cup celery, chopped
1 tsp cumin
4 cups water

---

1. Heat the oil in a large pan over a medium high-heat.
2. Add the leeks, garlic and cauliflower and sweat for 5-10 minutes (don't let them brown).
3. Add the celery and cumin and cook for another 5 minutes.
4. Add the water to the pan and bring to a boil.
5. Lower the heat and simmer for 15-20 minutes or until celery is soft.
6. Remove from heat and allow to cool before blending in a food processor or liquidizer.
7. Return to the pan and warm through.
8. Serve with a sprinkle of black pepper.

Per Serving: Calories 152
Protein 1 g
Carbohydrates 3 g
Fat 7 g
Sodium 5 mg
Potassium 59 mg
Phosphorus 34 mg

Mediterranean Vegetable Soup

SERVES 4 / PREP TIME: 5 MINUTES / COOK TIME: 30 MINUTES

Hearty, chunky soup.

---

1 tbsp extra-virgin olive oil
1 red onion, diced
2 garlic cloves, minced
1 zucchini, diced
1 cup eggplant, diced
1 red pepper, diced
4 cups water
1 tbsp oregano
1 tsp black pepper

---

1. Soak the vegetables in warm water prior to use.
2. In a large pot, add the oil, chopped onion and minced garlic.
3. Sweat for 5 minutes on a low heat.
4. Add the other vegetables to the onions and cook for 7-8 minutes.
5. Add the water to the pan and bring to a boil on a high heat.
6. Stir in the oregano, reduce the heat, and simmer for a further 20 minutes or until thoroughly cooked through.
7. Season with pepper to serve.

Per Serving: Calories 152
Protein 1 g
Carbohydrates 6 g
Fat 3 g
Sodium 3 mg
Potassium 229 mg
Phosphorus 45 mg

Renal Diet French Onion Soup

SERVES 4 / PREP TIME: 10 MINUTES / COOK TIME: 40 MINUTES

Amazing!

---

1 tbsp olive oil
3 onions, peeled and thinly sliced
1 tsp brown sugar
2 garlic cloves, minced
1 tbsp plain flour
1 cup low-sodium beef stock, hot
2 cups water
1 slice of white bread, cubed into croutons

---

1. Add the oil in a saucepan (with a lid) over a medium heat.
2. Sweat the onions for 2 minutes before adding the lid and leaving for 5-7 minutes until tender.
3. Remove the lid and sprinkle over the sugar.
4. Stir continuously for a few minutes until onions are golden brown and caramelized.
5. Now add the garlic and flour and stir.
6. Turn up the heat slightly.
7. Slowly add the beef stock and water whilst stirring.
8. Cover and simmer for 20 minutes.
9. Meanwhile, toast or grill the croutons.
10. Serve the soup with croutons and enjoy!

Per Serving: Calories 152
Protein 1 g
Carbohydrates 3 g
Fat 7 g
Sodium 5 mg
Potassium 59 mg
Phosphorus 29 mg

SIDES, SALADS, SNACKS & SAUCES

Pear & Brie Salad

SERVES 4 /   PREP TIME: 5 MINUTES /   COOK TIME: NA

Serve alone for lunch or as a refreshing side salad.

1/4 cucumber
/2 cup canned pears, juices drained
1 cup arugula
1/4 cup brie, chopped

1/2 lemon
1 tbsp olive oil

---

1. Peel and dice the cucumber.
2. Dice the pear.
3. Wash the arugula.
4. Combine salad in a serving bowl and crumble the brie over the top.
5. Whisk the olive oil and lemon juice together.
6. Drizzle over the salad.
7. Season with a little black pepper to taste and serve immediately.

Per Serving: Calories 54
Protein 1 g
Carbohydrates 12 g
Fat 7 g
Sodium 57mg
Potassium 115 mg
Phosphorus 67 mg

Herby Red Pepper Pasta Salad

SERVES 4 / PREP TIME: 5 MINUTES / COOK TIME: 20 MINUTES

This cooled pasta dish is delicious on the side of a juicy burger!

2 cups pasta
1 red bell pepper, finely diced
1/2 cucumber, finely diced
1/4 red onion, finely sliced
1 tsp black pepper
2 tbsp extra virgin olive oil
1 tsp dried tarragon
1 tsp dried oregano

1. Bring a pan of water (5 cups) to the boil before adding the pasta for 15-20 minutes or according to package directions.
2. Drain and allow pasta to cool before combining the rest of the raw ingredients and mixing well.
3. Serve right away or cover and refrigerate for 2-3 days.

Per Serving: Calories 188
Protein 4g
Carbohydrates 25 g
Fat 7 g
Sodium 2 mg
Potassium 143 mg
Phosphorus 57 mg

Carrot & Cilantro Coleslaw

SERVES 2 / PREP TIME: 5 MINUTES / COOK TIME: 5 MINUTES

A crunchy, healthy snack.

---

1 carrot, peeled and finely sliced
1 lemon, juice
1 tbsp fresh cilantro, finely chopped
1 tbsp extra virgin olive oil
Pinch of black pepper

---

1. Soak carrot slices in warm water for 5-10 minutes.
2. Boil a pan of water (3 cups) on a high heat and add the carrot slices for 30 seconds.
3. Drain and rinse with cold water.
4. Allow to cool.
5. Combine with the rest of the ingredients, cover and cool in the refrigerator before serving.

Per Serving: Calories 62
Protein 0g
Carbohydrates 5 g
Fat 7 g
Sodium 35 mg
Potassium 26 mg
Phosphorus 3 mg

Kidney-Friendly Chips

SERVES 4 / PREP TIME: 5 MINUTES / COOK TIME: 50 MINUTES

You'll love these healthy chips!

---

1 tbsp extra virgin olive oil
4 parsnips, peeled and sliced
1 tsp black pepper
1 tsp thyme

1 tsp chili flakes

---

1. Heat oven to 375°f/190°c/Gas Mark 5.
2. Grease a baking tray with the olive oil.
3. Add the parsnip slices in a thin layer.
4. Sprinkle over the thyme and chili slices and toss to coat.
5. Bake for 40-50 minutes (turning half way through to ensure even crispiness!)

Per Serving: Calories 62
Protein 0g
Carbohydrates 5 g
Fat 3 g
Sodium 7 mg
Potassium 115 mg
Phosphorus 112 mg

Bulgur & Roasted Peppers

SERVES 4 / PREP TIME: 10 MINUTES / COOK TIME: 20 MINUTES

The roasted Mediterranean flavors taste delicious with the bulgur.

1/2 cup dry bulgur
2 red bell peppers
2 lemon
1 tsp black pepper
1 tsp dried oregano
1 tsp mixed herbs
1 garlic clove

---

1. Soak the peppers in warm water prior to preparing.
2. Preheat the grill/broiler to a medium heat.
3. Wash the bulgur before adding to a bowl.
4. Pour 1/2 cup boiling water over the bulgur, cover and leave to sit for 30 minutes.
5. Drain any excess liquid from the bulgur.
6. Slice the red peppers into thin strips, drizzle with olive oil and sprinkle with herbs and pepper.
7. Throw in the garlic cloves whole and toss to coat.
8. Pour onto a baking tray and place under the grill for 15-20 minutes.
9. Turn over half way through.
10. Serve the red peppers, once soft and lightly char-grilled on top of the bulgur.
11. Add a little extra olive oil and lemon juice to the bulgur mixture.
12. Serve!

Per Serving: Calories 84
Protein 3g
Carbohydrates 18 g
Fat 3 g
Sodium 8 mg
Potassium 211 mg
Phosphorus 28 mg

Spaghetti Squash Puree

SERVES 8 / PREP TIME: 10 MINUTES / COOK TIME: 45 MINUTES

So easy to cook up and provides a real energy boost!

---

1 spaghetti squash (approx. 4 cups)
1 tsp chili flakes
3 tbsp parsley, finely chopped
1 tbsp extra virgin olive oil

---

1. Pre-heat the oven to 375°F/190 °C/Gas Mark 5.
2. Cut squash in half lengthways.
3. Place each side into a large oven dish (skin up).
4. Pour half a cup of water into the dish.
5. Bake for 45 minutes or until tender .
6. Remove from the oven and allow to cool.
7. Flake with a fork to shred the flesh into a bowl.
8. Stir in the chili flakes, parsley and olive oil.
9. Blend in a food processor until smooth.
10. Serve on your favorite salad or with your favorite meat.

Per Serving: Calories 32
Protein 0 g
Carbohydrates 4 g
Fat 2 g
Sodium 16 mg
Potassium 71 mg
Phosphorus 13 mg

Mexican Rice

SERVES 4 / PREP TIME: 5 MINUTES / COOK TIME: 25 MINUTES

A burst of flavor!

---

1 cup low-sodium chicken broth
1 cup water
1 cup uncooked white rice
1 tbsp extra virgin olive oil
1 red onion, chopped
1 red pepper, finely diced
1 lemon
1 tbsp cilantro, chopped

---

1. Add the stock, water and rice into a saucepan and boil over a high heat.
2. Once boiling, reduce the heat and simmer for 25 minutes until rice is cooked and the liquid is nearly absorbed.
3. Meanwhile, heat the oil in a skillet on a medium heat and sauté the onion until soft.
4. Add the peppers and cook for another 10 minutes.
5. Stir the onions and peppers into the rice and then squeeze in the lemon juice and top with cilantro to serve.

Per Serving: Calories
Protein 4 g
Carbohydrates 12 g
Fat 3 g
Sodium 9 mg
Potassium 9 mg
Phosphorus 22 mg

Lemony Green Beans

SERVES 4 / PREP TIME: 5 MINUTES / COOK TIME: 20 MINUTES

An amazing snack or tapas dish.

---

1 cup green beans
1 tbsp unsalted butter
1 lemon
Pinch black pepper

---

1. Steam the green beans over a high heat for 15-20 minutes or until soft.
2. Drain and place to one side to cool.
3. Heat the butter in a small pan until melted.
4. Whisk in the lemon juice.
5. Pour the lemon butter over the green beans, cover and allow to set the fridge for 30 minutes.
6. Serve with a pinch of black pepper.

Per Serving: Calories 34
Protein 0 g
Carbohydrates 2 g
Fat 2 g
Sodium 2 mg
Potassium 60 mg
Phosphorus 10 mg

Chili Sauce

SERVES 5 / PREP TIME: 5 MINUTES / COOK TIME: 20 MINUTES

Spice up fish, meat or vegetables!

2 tbsp canola oil
1 tbsp all-purpose white flour
1/4 cup tarragon vinegar
1/4 onion, finely diced
1 cup water
2 tsp dry mustard
1 tsp chili powder

1. Mix the oil and flour to form a paste before adding in the rest of the ingredients and pouring in to a pan.
2. Cook the mixture for 15-20 minutes over a low heat until it starts to thicken.
3. Remove from the heat and allow to cool or serve immediately hot.

Per Serving: Calories 70
Protein 0 g
Carbohydrates 2 g
Fat 5 g
Sodium 2 mg
Potassium 58 mg
Phosphorus 10 mg

Arugula Pesto

SERVES 5 / PREP TIME: 5 MINUTES / COOK TIME: NA

Delicious pesto dip, pasta sauce or salad dressing.

5 tbsp fresh basil
1 cup arugula
1 cup baby spinach
1 tsp black pepper
1/4 cup extra virgin olive oil
2 garlic cloves
1 lemon, juiced
1/4 cup brie (optional)

1. Blend all ingredients in a food processor or a blender to reach required texture - chunky for a rustic feel or smooth as a dressing.
2. Store in an airtight container in the fridge for 3-4 days.
3. Can be added to pasta for a delicious sauce, used as a dip with your favorite bread and served over a salad.

Per Serving: Calories 132
Protein 1 g
Carbohydrates 0 g
Fat 13 g
Sodium 50 mg
Potassium 36 mg
Phosphorus 51 mg

Brie & Beetroot Salad

SERVES 2 / PREP TIME: 5 MINUTES / COOK TIME: N/A

Amazing

1/2 cup brie
1 cup baby spinach leaves, washed
1/2 cup canned beets, juices drained &
sliced
Pinch black pepper
1 tbsp olive oil
1/4 cucumber, peeled and diced

---

1. Chop the brie into bite-size pieces.
2. Add all of the ingredients to a salad bowl and toss.
3. Serve right away.

Hint: If preparing the salad in advance, wait until just before serving to dress with olive oil or the salad will wilt.

Per Serving: Calories 283
Protein 14 g
Carbohydrates 3 g
Fat 23 g
Sodium 483 mg
Potassium 394 mg
Phosphorus 241 mg

Eggplant Dip

SERVES 4 / PREP TIME: 5 MINUTES / COOK TIME: 30 MINUTES

Homemade Baba Ganoush!

---

2 eggplants (approx. 4 cups)
2 tbsp extra virgin olive oil
2 garlic cloves, minced
1/2 onion. finely diced
1 tsp cumin
1 tsp turmeric
1 tbsp parsley
Pinch black pepper

---

1. Preheat the broiler/grill to a medium heat.
2. Slice the eggplants in half and add to a baking tray.
3. Drizzle over 1 tbsp olive oil and sprinkle over a pinch a black pepper.
4. Place under the grill for 15-20 minutes or until eggplants are soft and lightly grilled.
5. Now heat 1 tbsp oil in a skillet over a medium-high heat.
6. Add onions and sauté for 5 minutes or until soft.
7. Now add the cumin, followed by the turmeric and stir to release the aromas.
8. Turn the heat right down.
9. Now remove the eggplant and allow to cool slightly before scooping out the flesh.
10. Roughly chop with a sharp knife and add to the pan with the onions.
11. Sauté for 10 minutes and remove from the heat.
12. Allow to cool before blending in a food processor and adding parsley and black pepper.
13. Enjoy as a healthy dip.

Per Serving: Calories 70
Protein 2 g
Carbohydrates 9 g
Fat 3 g
Sodium 4 mg
Potassium 269 mg
Phosphorus 20 mg

Char-Grilled Veg Salad

SERVES 4 / PREP TIME: 5 MINUTES / COOK TIME: 20 MINUTES

Another delicious side dish.

---

1 eggplant, sliced (approx. 2 cups
2 tbsp olive oil
1 zucchini, peeled & sliced
2 diced red bell peppers, sliced
1/2 cup spinach leaves, washed
Pinch of pepper

---

1. Pre-heat a griddle pan over a high heat and add the eggplant slices for 10 minutes, turning over half way through, until lightly charred.
2. Remove from the pan and place to one side.
3. Now add a little live oil and the zucchini and pepper slices to the griddle pan.
4. Repeat above.
5. Mix all of the ingredients together with the spinach leaves.
6. Toss together and serve with a pinch of black pepper.

Per Serving: Calories 79
Protein 0 g
Carbohydrates 3 g
Fat 6 g
Sodium 4 mg
Potassium 215 mg
Phosphorus 54 mg

Homemade White Sauce

SERVES 5 / PREP TIME: 5 MINUTES / COOK TIME: 20 MINUTES

A low sodium alternative to shop-bought white sauces.

---

1 tbsp unsalted butter
1/4 cup all purpose white flour
3/4 cup rice milk (un-enriched)
1/4 cup brie if tolerated
1 tsp white pepper
1 tsp black pepper

---

1. Heat a small saucepan over a medium heat.
2. Add the butter to the pan.
3. Allow the butter to melt before gradually adding the flour.
4. Continue to stir until a smooth paste is formed.
5. Add the milk and stir thoroughly for 10 minutes until the lumps dissolve.
6. Add the cheese (optional) and stir for a further 5 minutes.
7. Turn off the heat and serve immediately.

Per Serving: Calories 79
Protein 2 g
Carbohydrates 4 g
Fat 6 g
Sodium 90 mg
Potassium 18 mg
Phosphorus 56 mg

Crab & Scallion Salad

SERVES 4 / PREP TIME: 5 MINUTES / COOK TIME: NA

A chunky salad on the side.

8oz crab meat
Juice of 1 lemon
Pinch of pepper
1 cup arugula, washed
1/4 cup scallions, washed and sliced
1 tbsp of olive oil

---

1. Mix the crab meat and lemon juice together.
2. Season with pepper and place to one side.
3. Into a salad bowl, add the arugula and scallions.
4. Drizzle with the olive oil and toss to coat.
5. Mix the crab meat with the salad and serve.

Per Serving: Calories 81
Protein 9 g
Carbohydrates 0 g
Fat 4 g
Sodium 286 mg
Potassium 197 mg
Phosphorus 86 mg

THE
RENAL SLOW COOKER COOKBOOK

with
50
DELICIOUS & HEARTY RENAL DIET RECIPES THAT PRACTICALLY COOK THEMSELVES

BREAKFAST

Easy Morning Slow Cooked Oats

SERVES 4 / PREP TIME: 5 MINUTES / COOK TIME: 7-8 HOURS

A brilliant bowl of energy to keep you up and running until lunch.

---

1 cup of jumbo oats
4 cups of almond milk (unenriched)
1 tsp. of ground cinnamon
To serve: 1 cup of raspberries

---

1. Heat your slow cooker.
2. Find a sturdy ceramic bowl that fits nicely in the cooker.
3. Put the oats in the bowl and pour the milk on top.
4. Sprinkle in the cinnamon.
5. Place the bowl in the slow cooker on its lowest setting
6. Cook overnight for 7-8 hours.
7. To serve, stir and add a drop more milk or water to your desired consistency.
8. Add the raspberries on top and enjoy.

Per Serving: Calories: 187
- Protein: 4g
- Carbohydrates: 33g
- Fat: 4g
- Cholesterol: 0mg
- Sodium: 159mg
- Potassium: 247mg
- Phosphorus: 112mg
- Calcium: 484mg
- Fiber: 5g

Soft & Spicy Vegetarian Enchiladas

SERVES 4 / PREP TIME: 10 MINUTES / COOK TIME: 2-3 HOURS

These soft and zingy enchiladas are filling, nutritious and great for sharing.

---

4 whole wheat tortillas
2 large egg whites
1 ½ cups of almond milk (unenriched)
(Optional) 1 red chili, de-seeded and
finely chopped
1 yellow bell pepper, chopped
¾ cup of sliced scallions

2 tbsp. of chopped fresh cilantro
1 tbsp. of finely chopped chives
1 cup of frozen peas

---

1. Spray the inside of your slow cooker with cooking spray.
2. Place two of the tortillas in the bottom of the slow cooker.
3. Using a fork beat the egg whites, milk and chili in a small bowl.
4. Keep 2 tbsp. of chopped bell pepper and 2 tbsp. of scallions set aside for later.
5. Tip the remaining bell pepper and scallions onto the tortillas.
6. Use the final two tortillas to cover it all up.
7. Pour the egg mixture over the top.
8. Cover with foil or baking paper and cook on a Low heat setting for 4 to 5 hours or on High heat setting 2 to 3 hours or until the centre is set.
9. Sprinkle with the rest of the bell pepper, scallions, cilantro and chives.
10. Remove the foil before serving by loosening the edges with a knife.

Per Serving: Calories: 180
Protein: 8g
Carbohydrates: 28g
Fat: 4g
Cholesterol: 0mg
Sodium: 293mg
Potassium: 309mg
Phosphorus: 173mg
Calcium: 201mg
Fiber: 7g

Light & Fluffy Frittata

SERVES 4 / PREP TIME: 10 MINUTES / COOK TIME: 4-5 HOURS

Light, healthy and full of flavor. Serve as a side or with a generous salad helping.

1 tsp. olive oil
1 cup of baby spinach
1 red bell pepper, finely diced
¼ cup of green onions, sliced
¼ cup of brie (optional, broken into small pieces)
1 tsp. of basil
3 large egg whites
1 tsp. of black pepper

1. Wash the spinach in a colander and pat it dry with a paper towel.
2. Lightly oil the inside of the slow cooker.
3. Add the red pepper, green onions and baby spinach to the cooker.
4. Beat the eggs vigorously with a fork and stir in the basil.
5. Pour in the mix and stir.
6. Sprinkle on the brie (optional).
7. Cook on the lowest setting for 1-2 hours or until the frittata is set and the brie is melted.
8. Serve hot.

Per Serving: Calories: 66
Protein: 5g
Carbohydrates: 3g
Fat: 4g
Cholesterol: 9mg
Sodium: 144mg
Potassium: 184mg
Phosphorus: 35mg
Calcium: 35mg
Fiber: 1g

Creamy Buckwheat & Plum Porridge

Smooth, warm and sweet with notes of spice.

5 cups of almond milk (un-enriched)
1 ½ cups buckwheat groats
2 tbsp. ground cinnamon
1 cup of plums, pitted and sliced

1. Add the almond milk to the slow cooker.
2. Pour in the buckwheat, cinnamon and sliced plum pieces.
3. Cook gently overnight on the lowest setting for 6-10 hours.
4. It's that simple!

Per Serving: Calories: 163
Protein: 4g
Carbohydrates: 34g
Fat: 2g
Cholesterol: 0mg
Sodium: 101mg
Potassium: 207mg
Phosphorus: 84mg
Calcium: 316mg
Fiber: 4g

Golden Broccoli Frittata

SERVES 12 / PREP TIME: 10 MINUTES / COOK TIME: 5 -7 HOURS

This frittata is hearty and delicious with a little bit of kick.

4 large egg whites
½ cup of coconut milk (unenriched)
1 tsp. of Dijon mustard
1 cup of scallions, chopped

½ tsp. of black pepper
1 head of broccoli, finely chopped
1 small white onion, diced
2 carrots, grated

1. Lightly oil your slow cooker with a little cooking spray.
2. Lightly beat together the egg whites, milk, dry mustard, scallions and pepper.
3. Place 1/3 of the broccoli in an even layer in the slow cooker.
4. Top with 1/3 of the onion and ½ of the carrot.
5. Repeat the layers two more times.
6. Pour the egg mixture over the top.
7. Cook on Low for 5-7 hours, or until eggs are set and the top is golden brown.
8. Share and serve with a crisp green salad.

Per Serving: Calories: 54
Protein: 3g
Carbohydrates: 6g
Fat: 3g
Cholesterol: 0mg
Sodium: 70mg
Potassium: 249mg
Phosphorus: 54mg
Calcium: 34mg
Fiber: 3g

MEAT

Mouthwatering Beef & Chilli Stew

SERVES 6 / PREP TIME: 15 MINUTES / COOK TIME: 7 HOURS

This is a rich, steaming stew with tender beef and sweet spices.

1/2 medium red onion, thinly sliced into half moons
1/2 tbsp. vegetable oil
10oz of flat cut beef brisket, whole
½ cup low sodium stock
¾ cup water
½ tbsp. honey
½ tbsp. chili powder
½ tsp. smoked paprika
½ tsp. dried thyme
1 tsp. black pepper
1 tbsp. corn starch

1. Throw the sliced onion into the slow cooker first.
2. Add a splash of oil to a large hot skillet and briefly seal the beef on all sides.
3. Remove the beef from skillet and place in the slow cooker.
4. Add the stock, water, honey and spices to the same skillet that you cooked the beef in.
5. Loosen the browned bits from bottom of pan with spatula. (Hint: These brown bits at the bottom are called the fond.)
6. Allow juice to simmer until the volume is reduced by about half.
7. Pour the juice over beef in the slow cooker.
8. Set slow cooker on Low and cook for approximately 7 hours.
9. Take the beef out of the slow cooker and onto a platter.
10. Shred it with two forks.
11. Pour the remaining juice into a medium saucepan. Bring to a simmer.
12. Whisk the cornstarch with two tbsp. of water.
13. Add to the juice and cook until slightly thickened.
14. For a thicker sauce, simmer and reduce the juice a bit more before adding cornstarch.
15. Pour the sauce over the meat and serve.

Per Serving: Calories: 128
Protein: 13g
Carbohydrates: 6g
Fat: 6g
Cholesterol: 39mg
Sodium: 228mg
Potassium: 202mg
Phosphorus: 119mg
Calcium: 16mg
Fiber: 1g

Beef & Three Pepper Stew

SERVES 6 / PREP TIME: 15 MINUTES / COOK TIME: 6 HOURS

Colorful and delicious, and perfect with a nice crusty white bread.

10oz of flat cut beef brisket, whole
1 tsp. of dried thyme
1 tsp. of black pepper
1 clove garlic
½ cup of green onion, thinly sliced
½ cup low sodium chicken stock
2 cups water

1 large green bell pepper, sliced
1 large red bell pepper, sliced
1 large yellow bell pepper, sliced
1 large red onion, sliced

---

1. Combine the beef, thyme, pepper, garlic, green onion, stock and water in a slow cooker.
2. Leave it all to cook on High for 4-5 hours until tender.
3. Remove the beef from the slow cooker and let it cool.
4. Shred the beef with two forks and remove any excess fat.
5. Place the shredded beef back into the slow cooker.
6. Add the sliced peppers and the onion.
7. Cook on High for 45 to 60 minutes until the vegetables are tender.

Per Serving: Calories: 132
Protein: 14g
Carbohydrates: 9g
Fat: 5g
Cholesterol: 39mg
Sodium: 179mg
Potassium: 390mg
Phosphorus: 141mg
Calcium: 33mg
Fiber: 2g

Sticky Pulled Beef Open Sandwiches

SERVES 5 / PREP TIME: 15 MINUTES / COOK TIME: 5 HOURS

These make a brilliant treat for barbecues with a rich, smoky taste.

½ cup of green onion, sliced
2 garlic cloves
2 tbsp. of fresh parsley
2 large carrots
7oz of flat cut beef brisket, whole
1 tbsp. of smoked paprika
1 tsp. dried parsley
1 tsp. of brown sugar
½ tsp. of black pepper
2 tbsp. of olive oil
¼ cup of red wine

8 tbsp. of cider vinegar
3 cups of water
5 slices white bread
1 cup of arugula to garnish

1. Finely chop the green onion, garlic and fresh parsley.
2. Grate the carrot.
3. Put the beef in to roast in a slow cooker.
4. Add the chopped onion, garlic and remaining ingredients, leaving the rolls, fresh parsley and arugula to one side.
5. Stir in the slow cooker to combine.
6. Cover and cook on Low for 8 to 10 hours, or on High for 4 to 5 hours until tender. (Hint: Test for tenderness by pressing into the meat with a fork.)
7. Remove the meat from the slow cooker.
8. Shred it apart with two forks.
9. Return the meat to the broth to keep it warm until ready to serve.
10. Lightly toast the bread and top with shredded beef, arugula, fresh parsley and ½ spoon of the broth.
11. Serve.

Per Serving: Calories: 273
Protein: 15g
Carbohydrates: 20g
Fat: 11g
Cholesterol: 37mg
Sodium: 308mg
Potassium: 399mg
Phosphorus: 159mg
Calcium: 113mg
Fiber: 3g

Herby Beef Stroganoff & Fluffy Rice

SERVES 6 / PREP TIME: 15 MINUTES / COOK TIME: 5 HOURS

This dish is rich and indulgent with aromatic herbs.

½ cup onion
2 garlic cloves
9 oz of flat cut beef brisket, cut into 1" cubes
½ cup of reduced-sodium beef stock
1/3 cup red wine
½ tsp. dried oregano
¼ tsp. freshly ground black pepper

½ tsp. dried thyme
½ tsp. of saffron
½ cup almond milk (unenriched)
¼ cup all-purpose flour
1 cup of water
2 ½ cups of white rice

1. Chop up the onion and mince the garlic cloves.
2. Mix the beef, stock, wine, onion, garlic, oregano, pepper, thyme and saffron in your slow cooker.
3. Cover and cook on High until the beef is tender, for about 4-5 hours.
4. Combine the almond milk, flour and water.
5. Whisk together until smooth.
6. Add the flour mixture to the slow cooker.
7. Cook for another 15 to 25 minutes until the stroganoff is thick.
8. Cook the rice using the package instructions, leaving out salt.
9. Drain off the excess water.
10. Serve the stroganoff over the rice.

Per Serving: Calories: 241
Protein: 15g
Carbohydrates: 29g
Fat: 5g
Cholesterol: 39g
Sodium: 182mg
Potassium: 206mg
Phosphorus: 151mg
Calcium: 59mg
Fiber: 1g

Beef Brisket with a Herby Sauce

SERVES 5 / PREP TIME: 15 MINUTES / COOK TIME: 8 HOURS

Succulent, chunky beef with a flavorful herb-infused sauce.

---

1 cup of onion
2 garlic cloves
10oz of flat cut beef brisket, whole
1 tbsp. of oregano
2 tsp. of Dijon mustard
1/2 tsp. of dried dill
1/2 tsp. of black pepper
½ cup of mushrooms, sliced

1/4 cup all-purpose white flour
1/4 cup of low-sodium beef stock
1 ½ cups of water

---

1. Chop the onion and mince the garlic.
2. Cut the brisket into 1/4" thick slices.
3. Place the steak, garlic, onions, seasoning and mushrooms in the slow cooker.
4. Stir it all well.
5. In a small bowl, gradually add the stock to the flour, stirring often.
6. Whisk it together until it's fully blended and free of lumps.
7. Add the broth mixture and the water to the pot and stir them in.
8. Cover with the lid and cook on High for 1 hour.
9. Reduce to Low and cook for 7 to 8 hours or until steak is tender.
10. Turn the slow cooker off, and remove lid.
11. Let the beef mixture stand for 10 minutes before serving.

Per Serving: Calories: 130
Protein: 15g
Carbohydrates: 5g
Fat: 5g
Cholesterol: 44mg
Sodium: 193mg
Potassium: 199mg
Phosphorus: 134mg
Calcium: 19mg
Fiber: 1g

Chunky Beef & Potato Slow Roast

SERVES 12 / PREP TIME: 15 MINUTES / COOK TIME: 5-6 HOURS

Chunky, warm and delicious, especially with a little horseradish kick on the side.

3 cups of peeled potatoes, chunked
1 cup of onion
2 garlic cloves, chopped
1 ¼ pounds flat cut beef brisket, fat trimmed
2 of cups water
1 tsp. of chili powder

1 tbsp. of dried rosemary
For the sauce:
1 tbsp. of freshly grated horseradish
½ cup of almond milk (unenriched)
1 tbsp. lemon juice (freshly squeezed)
1 garlic clove, minced
A pinch of cayenne pepper

1. Double boil the potatoes to reduce their potassium content.
2. (Hint: Bring your potato to the boil, then drain and refill with water to boil again.)
3. Chop the onion and the garlic.
4. Place the beef brisket in slow cooker.
5. Combine water, chopped garlic, chili powder and rosemary
6. Pour the mixture over the brisket.
7. Cover and cook on High for 4-5 hours until the meat is very tender.
8. Drain the potatoes and add them to the slow cooker.
9. Turn heat to High and cook covered until the potatoes are tender.
10. Prepare the horseradish sauce by whisking together horseradish, milk, lemon juice, minced garlic and cayenne pepper.
11. Cover and refrigerate.
12. Serve your casserole with a dash of horseradish sauce on the side.

Per Serving: Calories: 199
Protein: 21g
Carbohydrates: 12g
Fat: 7g
Cholesterol: 63mg
Sodium: 282mg
Potassium: 317
Phosphorus: 191mg
Calcium: 23mg
Fiber: 1g

Beef & Bean Sprout Stew

SERVES 6 / PREP TIME: 15 MINUTES / COOK TIME: 6-8 HOURS

A warm dish with vibrant flavors and a melt-in-the-mouth texture.

---

2 medium carrots
2 green onions
2 celery stalks
1 medium green bell pepper, sliced
1 garlic clove
8 oz. of canned bean sprouts
8 oz. of canned water chestnuts
2 tbsp. of coconut oil
12oz lean casserole beef, cut into cubes
½ cup low-sodium beef stock

1 tbsp. brown sugar
1/4 cup white wine vinegar
1 red chili, finely diced
1 ½ cups of water
3 cups cooked white rice

---

1. Slice the carrots, green onions, celery and green pepper.
2. Crush the garlic. (Hint: Use the flat edge of a knife to do this easily.)
3. Rinse and slice the bamboo shoots and water chestnuts.
4. Heat the coconut oil in a skillet and just brown the beef all over.
5. Transfer the beef to the slow cooker.
6. Add all the ingredients except the water.
7. Stir, then cover and cook on Low for 6 to 8 hours.
8. Turn the slow cooker up to High.
9. Add the cold water to the slow cooker.
10. Stir it in to make it smooth, and leave the cooker lid slightly open.
11. Cook for a further 15 minutes.
12. Serve your dish over a bed of rice.

Per Serving: Calories: 267
Protein: 14g
Carbohydrates: 31g
Fat: 9g
Cholesterol: 35mg
Sodium: 166mg
Potassium: 319mg
Phosphorus: 148mg
Calcium: 41mg
Fiber: 3g

Beef One-Pot Slow Roast

SERVES 8 / PREP TIME: 15 MINUTES / COOK TIME: 4-5 HOURS

A hot, hearty one-pot roast for large gatherings or cold evenings.

---

1 tbsp. plain flour
1 pound of boneless beef chuck or rump
roast
1 tbsp. of olive oil
¼ cup leek, sliced
2 garlic cloves, minced
½ cup rutabaga, peeled and cubed
½ tsp. of dried thyme
1/2 tsp. of dried parsley
1 ½ cups water
¼ cup of carrots, sliced

---

1. First, dust the beef in flour.
2. In a hot oiled skillet, brown the meat on all sides.
3. Add the onions, then cover and cook on Low for 15 minutes.
4. Add the garlic, rutabaga, herb seasoning and 2 cups of water.
5. Add to the slow cooker and simmer on a medium heat for 3 ½ to 4 hours, until the meat is tender.
6. Finally, add in the carrots and cook for an additional 30 minutes.

Per Serving: Calories: 100
Protein: 12g
Carbohydrates: 2.5g
Fat: 4g
Cholesterol: 35.5mg
Sodium: 25.5mg
Potassium: 149mg
Phosphorus: 82.5mg
Calcium: 19mg
Fiber: 0.5g

Smoky Turkey Chili

SERVES 8 / PREP TIME: 5 MINUTES / COOK TIME: 45 MINUTES

Succulent, smoky and mildly spiced. A perfect blend to sizzle your taste buds.

12oz lean ground turkey
1/2 red onion, chopped
2 cloves garlic, crushed and chopped
½ tsp. of smoked paprika
½ tsp. of chili powder
½ tsp. of dried thyme

¼ cup reduced-sodium beef stock
½ cup of water
1 ½ cups baby spinach leaves, washed
3 wheat tortillas

1. Brown the ground beef in a dry skillet over a medium-high heat.
2. Add in the red onion and garlic.
3. Sauté the onion until it goes clear.
4. Transfer the contents of the skillet to the slow cooker.
5. Add the remaining ingredients and simmer on Low for 30–45 minutes.
6. Stir through the spinach for the last few minutes to wilt.
7. Slice tortillas and gently toast under the broiler until slightly crispy.
8. Serve on top of the turkey chili.

Per Serving: Calories: 93.5
Protein: 8g
Carbohydrates: 3g
Fat: 5.5g
Cholesterol: 30.5mg
Sodium: 84.5mg
Potassium: 142.5mg
Phosphorus: 92.5mg
Calcium: 29mg
Fiber: 0.5g

Aromatic Spiced Chicken Curry

SERVES 4 / PREP TIME: 5 MINUTES / COOK TIME: 4-5 HOURS

Tender chicken with rich warming spices, incredibly easy and an impressive meal.

1 tbsp. of olive oil
1 onion, diced
1 tsp. of mild curry powder
1 carrot, peeled and diced
1 tsp. of turmeric
1 tsp. of allspice
1 tsp. of cumin

8oz of skinless chicken breast, diced
2 cups of water
A pinch of black pepper
2 cups of cooked white rice
2 tbsp. of fresh cilantro

1. Heat the oil in a large wok or skillet over a medium-high heat.
2. Add the onions and sauté for five minutes to soften (but not brown) them.
3. Now add the turmeric and stir briefly.
4. Next, add the allspice and stir.
5. Add the cumin and stir.
6. Transfer the onion mixture into the slow cooker.
7. Cook the chicken in the skillet until all sides are white.
8. Transfer to a slow cooker with the rest of the ingredients (minus the rice).
9. Cook for 4-5 hours on High or overnight on Low.
10. Serve your curry with white rice and a sprinkle of fresh cilantro.

Per Serving: Calories: 213
Protein: 15g
Carbohydrates: 25g
Fat: 5g
Cholesterol: 35mg
Sodium: 44mg
Potassium: 210mg
Phosphorus: 140mg
Calcium: 43mg
Fiber: 1g

Sticky Pork in Sweet & Sour Sauce

SERVES 4 / PREP TIME: 10 MINUTES / COOK TIME: 4 HOURS

A delicious blend of sweetness and acidity, with tender pork and light noodles.

8oz of lean pork roast, diced
1 cup of canned pineapple, juice drained
2 red bell peppers, diced
1 tsp. of soy sauce
1 tbsp. of tomato ketchup

1 tsp. of sage, dried
1 tbsp. red wine vinegar
2 cups of water
2 pak choy plants, washed and leaves pulled apart
2 cups of rice noodles
1 onion, chopped

---

1. Add all ingredients to a slow cooker, excluding the pak choy.
2. Leave to cook on High for 4-5 hours or on Low overnight.
3. 20 minutes before serving, add the rice noodles to a pan of boiling water and cook for 20 minutes or following package directions.
4. Add the pak choy leaves 10 minutes before serving.
5. Allow them to steam gently in the slow cooker.
6. In a deep dish, lay the noodles first, then spoon the pork and sauce on top.
7. Finally, add the steamed pak choy to finish.

Per Serving: Calories: 85
Protein: 9g
Carbohydrates: 9g
Fat: 1g
Cholesterol: 18mg
Sodium: 106mg
Potassium: 373mg
Phosphorus: 89mg
Calcium: 68mg
Fiber: 2g

Savory Pork & Bramley Apple Stew

SERVES 6 / PREP TIME: 10 MINUTES / COOK TIME: 8-10 HOURS

Soft, savory pork with the warm flavor of apple. A match made in heaven.

12oz of pork loin, whole
1 cup of Bramley apples, peeled and
cubed
A pinch of black pepper
1 tsp. of cloves
2 tbsp. of dried sage
4 cups of water

---

1. Rub the pork loin with the herbs and spices and place in the slow cooker.
2. Add the apple cubes and the water.
3. Add in the seasoning.
4. Cover and cook on Low for 8 to 10 hours.
5. Transfer the pork loin to a chopping board.
6. Leave it to rest for 5-10 minutes.
7. Carve the cooked loin into thick slices.
8. Serve the pork slices with the apple and the juices from the pot

Per Serving: Calories: 115
Protein: 15g
Carbohydrates: 5g
Fat: 4g
Cholesterol: 43mg
Sodium: 31mg
Potassium: 237mg
Phosphorus: 129mg
Calcium: 46mg
Fiber: 1g

Honey Mustard Marinated Pork Loin

SERVES 6 / PREP TIME: 10 MINUTES / COOK TIME: 4-5 HOURS

Sweet and tangy with tender vegetables and meltingly soft pork.

12oz of pork loin, boneless, fat-trimmed
and cubed
1 tbsp. of Dijon mustard
2 tbsp. of honey
2 tbsp. of coconut oil
1 medium white onion, roughly chopped
1 zucchini, roughly chopped
4 cups of water
1 tsp. of chili flakes
1 tsp. of dried sage
1 tsp. of ground nutmeg

---

1. Whisk together the honey, mustard and coconut oil.
2. Marinate the pork loin for at least 8 hours in the refrigerator.
3. Add the pork and remaining marinade to the slow cooker along with the vegetables.
4. Next, pour in the water and ensure the pork is well covered.
5. Sprinkle in the herbs and spices.
6. Cook on High for 4-5 hours.
7. Remove and serve steaming hot with white rice or rice noodles.

Per Serving: Calories: 134
Protein: 10g
Carbohydrates: 8g
Fat: 7g
Cholesterol: 29mg
Sodium: 60mg
Potassium: 235mg
Phosphorus: 100mg
Calcium: 29mg
Fiber: 1g

Cauliflower & Lamb Tagine

SERVES 5 / PREP TIME: 20 MINUTES / COOK TIME: 4-5 HOURS

The spices create a deep, authentic Moroccan flavor to the lamb with cauliflower to add a little crunch.

1 tbsp. of all-purpose flour
8oz of lean lamb, diced
1 tbsp. of olive oil
1 tbsp. of sweet paprika
1 tsp. cumin
1 tsp. of turmeric
1 red onion, diced
2 cups of cauliflower florets
4 cups water
4 white pita breads

1. In a shallow bowl with the flour, place the diced lamb.
2. Shake the bowl to dust the lamb.
3. Remove the lamb from the bowl.
4. Combine the spices in a measuring cup and evenly coat the floured lamb with the spices.
5. Heat the oil in a pan and then add the lamb cubes.
6. Brown on each side (5-10 minutes).
7. Transfer all the ingredients (minus the cauliflower) to the slow cooker.
8. Cook everything on High for 4-5 hours.
9. In the last 20 minutes, add the cauliflower florets and stir.
10. Lightly toast the pita breads when ready to serve.
11. Serve the tagine in a bowl with pita bread on the side for dipping.

Per Serving: Calories: 185
Protein: 14g
Carbohydrates: 17g
Fat: 7g
Cholesterol: 32mg
Sodium: 273mg
Potassium: 290mg
Phosphorus: 127mg
Calcium: 63mg
Fiber: 3g

Roasted Lamb with Mint & Garlic

SERVES 6 / PREP TIME: 15 MINUTES / COOK TIME: 5-6 HOURS

Lamb is at its best when rubbed with mint. Serve in thick slices for a succulent, tender roast.

10 oz. of lean lamb loin, boneless	2 cups carrots, peeled and roughly chopped
3 garlic cloves, whole	1 cup of water
1 tbsp. of olive oil	
2 tbsp. of fresh mint, finely chopped	
1 sheet of baking paper	
2 cups zucchini, roughly chopped	

1. Prepare the lamb by using a knife to make shallow carvings across the flesh.
2. Poke each garlic clove into the slices.
3. Mix the olive oil and mint to create a paste.
4. Rub this into the lamb.
5. Place the lamb in the slow cooker and cover baking paper.
6. Cook on high for 5-6 hours or until lamb is very soft.
7. In the last hour, add the carrots, zucchini and water.
8. Cook the vegetables until they're tender.
9. Serve hot with a drizzle of the lamb's lovely juices.

Per Serving: Calories: 153
Protein: 15g
Carbohydrates: 7g
Fat: 7g
Cholesterol: 44mg
Sodium: 223mg
Potassium: 420mg
Phosphorus: 147mg
Calcium: 44mg
Fiber: 2g

Kashmiri Spiced Lamb Curry

SERVES 6 / PREP TIME: 20 MINUTES / COOK TIME: 3 HOURS

Don't be put off by the long list of spices; they're worth it for the rich mellow flavor

---

2 red chilis, finely diced
1 tsp. cumin seeds
½ tbsp. fresh ginger, peeled and grated
3 cloves garlic, crushed
2 tbsp. of olive oil
1 cup white onions, sliced thinly

9oz lean lamb loin, washed, pat dry and cut into cubes
1 ½ cups almond milk (unenriched)
1/2 tsp. turmeric
1 tsp. cardamom pods, crushed slightly
1 ½ cups white rice
¼ cup chopped fresh cilantro

---

1. Grind the red chilis, cumin seeds, ginger and garlic together into a smooth paste using a blender or pestle and mortar.
2. Heat the oil in a pan over a medium heat and sauté the onions until golden.
3. Add the spice paste to the pan and stir until the oil separates from the mixture.
4. Now, add the lamb pieces and brown for 5 minutes whilst stirring.
5. Add the almond milk and turmeric and mix well.
6. Transfer to the slow cooker and add the star anise and cardamom pods.
7. Cook on a low heat for 2 hours until the lamb is very tender.
8. 20 minutes before serving, pour 6 cups of cold water to a pan.
9. Add the rice to the water and bring to a boil.
10. Turn down the heat and simmer for another 15 minutes.
11. Drain and return to pan with the lid on for 5 minutes to steam.
12. Serve with freshly steamed rice and garnish with fresh cilantro.

Per Serving: Calories: 204
Protein: 15g
Carbohydrates: 19g
Fat: 7g
Cholesterol: 40mg
Sodium: 214mg
Potassium: 379mg
Phosphorus: 133mg
Calcium: 139mg
Fiber: 1g

Roast Pork & Tangy Cabbage Slaw

SERVES 4 / PREP TIME: 20 MINUTES / COOK TIME: 8 HOURS

Lightly spiced pork, aromatic cloves and a crunchy, zesty slaw. Great for barbecues.

1 tsp. of nutmeg
1 tsp. of allspice
1 tbsp. of dried sage
1 tbsp. of olive oil
8oz of lean pork loin
1 tsp. of cloves
2 white of onions, chopped
2 cups of water
2 carrots, peeled and grated

1 cup of white cabbage, washed and grated or spiralized
1 lime, juiced

1. Mix nutmeg, allspice and sage with olive oil to form a marinade.
2. Coat the pork and marinate for as long as you can.
3. When ready to cook, evenly press the cloves into the pork.
4. Add the pork loin with the onions and water to the slow cooker.
5. Cook on Medium for 8 hours until the pork is very soft.
6. Meanwhile, prepare your slaw.
7. Mix the carrot and cabbage, and squeeze over the lime juice.
8. Cover and place in the fridge until you're ready to serve.
9. Remove the loin and slice generously.
10. Serve with the slaw, a helping of onions and a drizzle of the juices.
11. Don't forget to pick out the cloves before serving!

Per Serving: Calories: 129
Protein: 10g
Carbohydrates: 13g
Fat: 5g
Cholesterol: 23mg
Sodium: 25mg
Potassium: 343mg
Phosphorus: 109mg
Calcium: 60mg
Fiber: 3g

Chili Pork & Rice Noodles

SERVES 5 / PREP TIME:5 MINUTES / COOK TIME: 1.5 HOURS

Light rice noodles and chili infused pork, this is a dish to add to your go-to recipe list.

1 tbsp. olive oil
2 white onions, diced
2 garlic cloves, minced
1 red chili, finely diced
8oz lean ground pork
2 cups water
1 tsp. oregano
1 tsp. dried basil
1 tbsp. balsamic vinegar

2 cups of rice noodles
A pinch of black pepper

1. Heat the oil in a skillet over a medium-high heat.
2. Add the onions and sauté them for 5 minutes until soft.
3. Add in the garlic and chili and sauté for a further 5 minutes.
4. Add the ground pork and cook until its' browned (5-10 minutes).
5. Pour the pork mixture into the slow cooker
6. Add the water, herbs and vinegar.
7. The pork should be just covered but not swimming.
8. Cook on the High for 1 hour.
9. The sauce should be nice and thick at this point.
10. While waiting, prepare your pasta by following the package directions.
11. Serve the cooked spaghetti with a serving of pork chili and a pinch of sprinkled black pepper on top.

Per Serving: Calories: 286
Protein: 14g
Carbohydrates: 29g
Fat: 12g
Cholesterol: 42mg
Sodium: 200mg
Potassium: 351mg
Phosphorus: 153mg
Calcium: 54mg
Fiber: 2g

Roast Beef & Chunky Vegetable Stew

SERVES 8/ PREP TIME: 15 MINUTES / COOK TIME: 8-10 HOURS

Deliciously hearty and beautifully filling.

1 cup of rutabaga, peeled and cut into cubes
1 cup of potato, peeled and cut into cubes
1 cup of carrots, cut into 2-inch pieces
1 red onion, cut into wedges
3 cloves garlic, finely chopped

1 tbsp. of olive oil
16oz of flat cut beef brisket
1 tsp. of freshly ground pepper
1 cup of low sodium chicken stock
½ cup of water
3 tbsp. of chopped fresh parsley

1. Spray your slow cooker dish with a little cooking spray.
2. In the slow cooker, stir together the rutabaga, potato, carrots, onion and garlic.
3. In a large skillet, heat the oil over medium-high heat.
4. Sprinkle the beef with ground pepper and lay it in the skillet.
5. Cook until browned evenly on all sides.
6. Place the vegetables in the slow cooker.
7. Lay the beef on top.
8. Pour the stock and water over the beef.
9. Cover and cook on Low for 8 to 10 hours or until the beef is very tender.
10. Serve the beef along with the vegetables and the juices.
11. Garnish the top with a sprinkle of fresh parsley.

Per Serving: Calories: 151
Protein: 13g
Carbohydrates: 11g
Fat: 6g
Cholesterol: 36mg
Sodium: 101mg
Potassium: 373mg
Phosphorus: 140mg
Calcium: 33mg
Fiber: 2g

Ginger & Lemon Lamb with Noodles

SERVES 5 / PREP TIME: 10 MINUTES / COOK TIME: 2.5 HOURS

Delicate lamb with zesty flavors of lemon and ginger.

8oz lean lamb loin
1 tbsp. of coconut oil
1 tbsp. of fresh root ginger, finely sliced
4 garlic cloves
1 tbsp. of soft light brown sugar
Rind of 1 lemon
1 bunch of scallions

1 cup of pak choy, leaves separated
4 cups of rice noodles

---

1. Place the lamb in an oiled slow cooker dish.
2. Cook on High for 15 minutes to start.
3. Meanwhile, peel and slice the ginger and the garlic.
4. Add to the slow cooker with the sugar and lemon.
5. Cover the ingredients with water.
6. Cook on High for a further 15 minutes.
7. Reduce to Medium and cover the lamb with baking paper.
8. Cook for a further 2 hours or until the lamb is very tender.
9. Carve the lamb into nice thick slices.
10. Place the lamb on a warmed serving platter.
11. Cover it up and keep it warm in a low oven.
12. Roughly chop the scallions and thickly slice the pak choy.
13. Cook the noodles according to package directions.
14. Stir in the scallions and pak choy leaves.
15. Return to the boil and bubble, they only need a minute or so.
16. Serve the noodles immediately with the slices of lamb on top and the juices drizzled over.

Per Serving: Calories: 264
Protein: 15g
Carbohydrates: 33g
Fat: 7g
Cholesterol: 43mg
Sodium: 222mg
Potassium: 343mg
Phosphorus: 144mg
Calcium: 60mg
Fiber: 2g

POULTRY

Chicken & Squash Slow Roast

SERVES 8 / PREP TIME: 20 MINUTES / COOK TIME: 8-10 HOURS

This is a great winter warming dish for family gatherings or just some good comfort food.

3oz of all-purpose flour
1 tbsp. of coconut oil
10oz of boneless, skinless chicken breast, chopped
1 red onion, chopped
3 garlic cloves, finely chopped
1 tsp. of chili powder
1 spaghetti squash, cut into half (horizontally)
1 cup of low sodium chicken stock
1 cup of water

5 sprigs of fresh thyme (or 1 tbsp. dried)
3 bay leaves
A pinch of black pepper
2 tbsp. of chopped fresh parsley (optional)

1. Sprinkle the flour onto a plate.
2. Heat half of the oil in a skillet.
3. Dust the chicken pieces in the flour.
4. Cook the chicken for 4-5 minutes, or until browned all over. (Hint: You may need to brown the chicken a little at a time.)
5. Tip the chicken into the slow cooker.
6. Heat the remaining oil in a skillet and fry the onion until clear
7. Add in the garlic and cook for another 2-3 minutes.
8. Tip the onion mixture into the slow cooker too.
9. Add the chicken stock, thyme, chili powder and bay leaves to the slow cooker.
10. Stir everything together, pressing down so that everything is covered in liquid.
11. Press each half of the spaghetti squash into the mixture (skin side up).
12. Cook for 8-10 hours on Low.
13. Stir in the black pepper and parsley before serving.

Per Serving: Calories: 145
Protein: 15g
Carbohydrates: 13g
Fat: 4g
Cholesterol: 41mg
Sodium: 237mg
Potassium: 266mg
Phosphorus: 128mg
Calcium: 21mg
Fiber: 1g

Turmeric Curried Chicken

SERVES 6 / PREP TIME: 15 MINUTES / COOK TIME: 5 HOURS

Soft, juicy chicken with a delicious curry sauce with a little bit of a kick.

8oz skinless, boneless chicken breast
1 red bell pepper, chopped
1 yellow bell pepper, chopped
1 small white onion, sliced
1 fresh red chili pepper, de-seeded and finely chopped
2 cloves of garlic, minced
1 cup of low-sodium chicken stock
3 tbsp. of curry powder

1/4 tsp. of turmeric
1/2 cup almond milk (unenriched)
1 tsp. of cornstarch
2 cups white rice, cooked
2 tbsp. of fresh cilantro, chopped

---

1. Combine the chicken, peppers, onion, chili, garlic, stock, curry powder and turmeric in the slow cooker.
2. Cover and cook on Low for 8- 9 hours or on High for about 4½ hours.
3. In a small bowl, mix the almond milk and cornstarch until smooth.
4. Stir into chicken mixture.
5. If you're cooking on Low, turn up the heat to High now.
6. Cover and cook for 15 to 20 minutes more.
7. The sauce should be slightly thick by now.
8. Serve on white rice and sprinkle the with cilantro to finish.

Per Serving: Calories: 182
Protein: 15g
Carbohydrates: 25g
Fat: 3g
Cholesterol: 36mg
Sodium: 213mg
Potassium: 390mg
Phosphorus: 155mg
Calcium: 76mg
Fiber: 2g

Fennel & Ginger Chicken

SERVES 6 / PREP TIME: 1 MINUTES / COOK TIME: 2-3 HOURS

Fragrant fennel & ginger slow cooked chicken breasts.

12oz of skinless boneless chicken breast, diced
1/4 tsp. ground black pepper
1 bulb fennel, cored and cut into thin wedges
1 red bell pepper, de-seeded and diced
1 medium red onion, diced
3 cloves of garlic, minced
1 tsp. fresh or dried rosemary
1 tsp. of fresh or dried ginger (finely sliced if fresh)

½ cup reduced-sodium chicken stock
½ cup of water
1 tbsp. of dried oregano

---

1. Sprinkle the chicken pieces with ground pepper.
2. Place the chicken into the slow cooker.
3. Top with fennel, bell pepper, onion, garlic, rosemary and ginger.
4. Add the stock and water.
5. Cover and cook on Low for 5 to 6 hours or on High for 2½ to 3 hours.
6. Sprinkle each serving with oregano to finish.

Per Serving: Calories: 95
Protein: 15g
Carbohydrates: 4g
Fat: 2g
Cholesterol: 45mg
Sodium: 270mg
Potassium: 348mg
Phosphorus: 130mg
Calcium: 35mg
Fiber: 1g

Spanish-Style Chicken

SERVES 5 / PREP TIME: 5 MINUTES / COOK TIME: 3 ½ -4 HOURS

This blend of spices brings a smoky and intense flavor to the table.

10oz skinless, boneless chicken thighs, cut into cubes
2 large red onions, roughly chopped
1 garlic clove, minced
½ tsp. of dried oregano
¼ tsp. of ground black pepper
1 cup of reduced-sodium chicken stock

1 cup of water
1 medium red bell pepper, roughly chopped
1 tsp. of paprika
1 tsp. of cumin
2 cups of cooked white rice

1. In the slow cooker, combine the chicken, onion, garlic, oregano and black pepper.
2. Add in the stock and water.
3. Cover and cook on Low for 7 to 8 hours or on High for 3 ½ to 4 hours.
4. If using Low, turn the heat up to High at this point.
5. Stir in the red pepper, paprika and cumin.
6. Cover and cook for another 30 minutes.
7. Serve steaming hot with fluffy white rice.

Per Serving: Calories: 188
Protein: 11g
Carbohydrates: 29g
Fat: 3g
Cholesterol: 39mg
Sodium: 46mg
Potassium: 343mg
Phosphorus: 143mg
Calcium: 44mg
Fiber: 2g

Tender Spice-Rubbed Turkey Thighs

SERVES 4 / PREP TIME: 5 MINUTES / COOK TIME: 7-8 HOURS

Fragrant spices, juicy turkey and a tangy salsa on the side.

---

1 tsp. of cumin
1 tsp. of cinnamon
1 tsp. of chili powder
1 tsp. of dried oregano
1 garlic clove, minced
8oz of turkey thighs, skinless and boneless

A pinch of black pepper
1 red onion, soaked in warm water
1 lime, juiced
2 tbsp. of fresh cilantro, chopped

Mix the dry spices, herbs and minced garlic in a bowl to form a rub.

Rub the turkey thighs with the spice mix.

Place in the bottom of the slow cooker in a single layer.

Cook for 7-8 hours on a low setting.

Meanwhile, prepare your salsa. (Hint: Do this the night before and refrigerate for a better flavor.)

Finely dice the red onion and mix it with the fresh lime juice.

Remove the turkey thighs from the slow cooker.

Place them onto a chopping board.

Cut the thighs into slices.

Sprinkle the cilantro into the salsa before serving.

Serve on a plate with a helping of salsa.

Per Serving: Calories: 113
Protein: 15g
Carbohydrates: 8g
Fat: 3g
Cholesterol: 60mg
Sodium: 260mg
Potassium: 245mg
Phosphorus: 131mg
Calcium: 41mg
Fiber: 2g

Turkey & Lemon Rice Stew

SERVES 5 / PREP TIME: 15 MINUTES / COOK TIME: 6-7 HOURS

Tender turkey with a twist of lemon, and a salad to bring it all together with crunch.

---

1 tbsp. of olive oil
8oz of turkey breast tenderloins, skinless and boneless, diced
½ cup chopped celery
1/3 cup of chopped carrot
¼ cup of chopped red onion
1 cup of low sodium chicken stock
1 cup of water

1 tsp. of dried oregano
A pinch of black pepper
1.5 cups of white rice, rinsed and drained
1 lemon, juiced
1 cucumber, washed and sliced
1 cup of romaine lettuce or similar, washed
2 tbsp. of extra virgin olive oil

---

1. Heat the oil in a skillet over a medium heat.
2. Add in the turkey breast.
3. Cook for 3-5 minutes, stirring often until the turkey is brown.
4. Stir in the celery, carrot and onion.
5. Cook for 2 minutes, stirring occasionally.
6. Drain off the excess juices.
7. In the slow cooker, mix the turkey mixture and remaining ingredients except lemon, extra virgin olive oil, cucumber and lettuce.
8. Cover with the lid and cook on High for 30 minutes.
9. Reduce the heat to a Low.
10. Cook for 6-7 hours, or until the rice is tender and the liquid is absorbed.
11. Stir in the juice of half a lemon.
12. Slice the cucumber and lettuce for the side salad.
13. Whisk the remaining lemon juice and olive oil together.
14. Dress the salad with the lemon and oil dressing.
15. Serve on the side of your turkey.

Per Serving: Calories: 207
Protein: 12g
Carbohydrates: 20g
Fat: 9g
Cholesterol: 26mg
Sodium: 53mg
Potassium: 339mg
Phosphorus: 131mg
Calcium: 43mg
Fiber: 2g

Moroccan-Style Apricot Turkey Stew

SERVES 8 / PREP TIME: 5 MINUTES / COOK TIME: 3 ½ -4 HOURS

Rich spices, soft turkey and the sweetness of apricot come together for a delicious family meal.

4 carrots, peeled and sliced
2 large red onions, thinly sliced
12oz of turkey breast, skinless and boneless, diced
½ cup of canned apricots, drained and coarsely chopped
1 cup of low sodium chicken stock
2 tbsp. of all-purpose flour
2 tbsp. of lemon juice, freshly squeezed

2 cloves of garlic, minced
1 ½ tsp. of ground cumin
1 ½ tsp. of ground ginger
1 tsp. of ground nutmeg
¾ tsp. of ground black pepper
3 cups of cooked white rice
3 tbsp. of fresh cilantro, finely chopped

1. Add the carrots and onions into the slow cooker.
2. Add the diced turkey to cooker too, and top with the apricots.
3. In bowl, whisk the stock, flour, lemon juice, garlic, cumin, ginger, nutmeg and the ground black pepper.
4. Add the mixture to the cooker.
5. Cover and cook on Low for 6 ½ to 7 hours or on High for 3 ½ to 4 hours.
6. Serve the rice in bowls with the turkey and the sauce on top.
7. Garnish with cilantro to finish.

Per Serving: Calories: 189
Protein: 13g
Carbohydrates: 33g
Fat: 1g
Cholesterol: 24mg
Sodium: 45mg
Potassium: 371mg
Phosphorus: 144mg
Calcium: 45mg
Fiber: 3g

Garlic & Sesame Chicken

SERVES 4 / PREP TIME: 15 MINUTES / COOK TIME: 6-8 HOURS

A quick and delicious version of a classic Chinese dish.

---

2 carrots, peeled and sliced
2 green onions, finely chopped
4 celery stalks, sliced
2 garlic cloves, minced
2 tbsp. of sesame oil
8oz of boneless, skinless chicken breast, diced
1 cup of low-sodium chicken stock
1 tsp. of low-sodium soy sauce
1 tbsp. of Chinese five-spice
1 tsp. of fresh ginger, minced

⅓ cup of water
2 cups of snow peas
3 cups of cooked white rice
1 lime, juiced

---

1. Slice the carrots, green onions and celery.
2. Crush the garlic.
3. Heat the oil in a skillet and add the diced chicken.
4. Cook the chicken until it's nicely browned all over.
5. Transfer the chicken from the skillet to the slow cooker.
6. Add all the other ingredients (except the lime juice and snow peas).
7. Stir, then cover up and cook on a Low for 6 to 8 hours.
8. In the last 10 minutes, add the snow peas to the slow cooker.
9. Put on the lid slightly ajar to allow the peas to steam.
10. Serve the chicken and vegetables over rice with a squeeze of fresh lime.

Per Serving: Calories: 127
Protein: 11g
Carbohydrates: 8g
Fat: 6g
Cholesterol: 23mg
Sodium: 93mg
Potassium: 350mg
Phosphorus: 111mg
Calcium: 57mg
Fiber: 3g

Slow Cooked BBQ Chicken

SERVES 8 / PREP TIME: 5 MINUTES / COOK TIME: 6 HOURS

Sweet, smoky and melt-in-the-mouth with a tingle of spice.

16oz skinless, skinless boneless chicken breast fillets, whole
2 tbsp. of mustard
2 tsp. of lemon juice
1 garlic clove, finely grated
1/4 cup of brown sugar
1/2 tsp. of chili powder

1 tbsp. of tomato ketchup
4 white hamburger rolls, sliced in half
3 cups of arugula, washed

---

1. Place the chicken breasts into the bottom of the slow cooker.
2. In a bowl, stir together the mustard, lemon juice, garlic, brown sugar, chili powder and tomato ketchup.
3. Mix it together well.
4. Pour in the sauce, set the cooker to Low and cook for 6 hours.
5. Shred the chicken with two forks and cook for 30 more minutes.
6. Serve the chicken and sauce spooned onto each half of the hamburger bun with the arugula on top.

Per Serving: Calories: 141
Protein: 15g
Carbohydrates: 14g
Fat: 2g
Cholesterol: 35mg
Sodium: 160mg
Potassium: 177mg
Phosphorus: 121mg
Calcium: 56mg
Fiber: 1g

Slow Cooked Roast Chicken

SERVES 10 / PREP TIME: 20 MINUTES / COOK TIME: 4 HOURS 15 MINS

A classic roast. Juicy, indulgent and stuffed to perfection.

---

3 pounds of whole chicken, giblets removed
1 tsp. of olive oil
1 tsp. of ground black pepper
1 carrot, peeled and chopped
2 garlic cloves, whole
½ medium red onion, quartered
1 medium celery stalk, roughly chopped

¼ cup of white breadcrumbs
1 cup of broccoli florets

---

1. Trim any excess fat off the chicken.
2. In a food processor, mix everything but the chicken and broccoli.
3. This is for your stuffing.
4. Stuff the chicken cavity.
5. Place the whole chicken into the slow cooker.
6. Cook on High for 4 hours, until the thigh and leg easily pull away and the meat easily comes off the bones.
7. Remove the skin and discard.
8. Remove the meat from the bones and place to one side.
9. Weigh the meat before serving – you should serve only 2oz of chicken per person.
10. Prepare the broccoli by steaming for 10-15 minutes.
11. Serve the roasted chicken with the steamed broccoli.
12. (Hint: Allow the rest of the meat to cool before covering and placing in fridge for 2-3 days or freezer for 2-3 weeks.)
13. You can also use the stock from the slow cooker – simply sieve out any chunks and allow to cool. Repeat above.

Per Serving: Calories: 87   Fiber: 1g
Protein: 13.5g
Carbohydrates: 4g
Fat: 2g
Cholesterol: 40.5mg
Sodium: 224mg
Potassium: 248mg
Phosphorus: 115.5mg
Calcium: 25mg

VEGETARIAN AND VEGAN

Winter Spiced Squash Stew

SERVES 6 / PREP TIME: 15 MINUTES / COOK TIME: 6-7 HOURS

A Winter favorite with soft, sweet squash and warm flavors.

1 spaghetti squash
2 medium zucchini
1/2 cup of yellow bell pepper
1 cup of unsweetened canned pineapple, diced
½ cup of water
1 tsp. of allspice
2 ½ tbsp. of brown sugar substitute
1 tbsp. of unsalted butter

1. Cut the squashes down the middle (horizontally).
2. Dice the bell pepper into small pieces.
3. Placed the squash halves into the slow cooker (skin side up).
4. In a small bowl, mix the pepper, pineapple, ½ cup of water, allspice, brown sugar and melted butter.
5. Pour the mix into the slow cooker around the base of the squash.
6. Cover the squash and cook on a Low for 6-7 hours or until squash is tender.
7. Stir the pot gently to mix the ingredients well before serving.

Per Serving: Calories: 63
Protein: 1g
Carbohydrates: 10g
Fat: 3g
Cholesterol: 5mg
Sodium: 18mg
Potassium: 309mg
Phosphorus: 37mg
Calcium: 38mg
Fiber: 2g

Vegetable Stew with Mediterranean Spices

SERVES 4 / PREP TIME: 10 MINUTES / COOK TIME: 1-2 HOURS

Soft and sweet with a beautiful blend of spices.

---

1 zucchini, sliced
2 red bell peppers, sliced
2 eggplants, diced
2 medium white onions, diced
3 cups of water
1 cup of low sodium vegetable stock (optional)
1 tsp. of dried thyme
1 tsp. of nutmeg
1 tsp. of paprika
1 tbsp. of cider vinegar
1 tbsp. of ground black pepper
1 tbsp. all-purpose flour
2 garlic cloves, peeled and halved
2 cups white rice

2 tbsp. fresh basil, chopped

---

1. Wash and roughly chop the vegetables into large pieces.
2. Bring the water to a boil in a saucepan.
3. Mix the flour with the boiled water until the lumps dissolve.
4. Now add all the ingredients into the slow cooker.
5. Cook on Low for 1-2 hours or until the vegetables are soft and the sauce is thickened.
6. Serve with fluffy white rice and a garnish of fresh basil.

Per Serving: Calories: 154
Protein: 4g
Carbohydrates: 34g
Fat: 1g
Cholesterol: 0mg
Sodium: 132mg
Potassium: 380mg
Phosphorus: 85mg
Calcium: 63mg
Fiber: 4

Chunky Root Vegetable Roast

SERVES 6 / PREP TIME: 10 MINUTES / COOK TIME: 3-4 HOURS

Best served steaming hot with helping of crusty white bread on the side.

1 rutabaga, peeled and cubed
2 large carrots, peeled and cubed
2 turnips, peeled and cubed
2 cups of water
1 tbsp. of all-purpose flour
1 garlic clove, minced

1 cup of low sodium vegetable stock
(optional)
2 tbsp. dried oregano
1 tbsp. black pepper
1 loaf of crusty white bread

1. Peel and chop the rutabaga, carrots and turnips into cubes.
2. Boil the water and stir in the flour until lumps have dissolved.
3. Add all of the remaining ingredients to the slow cooker.
4. Cook on a Low 3-4 hours or until vegetables are tender.
5. Serve in hearty bowls.
6. Toast the bread and serve it on the side of the casserole.
7. Dip and enjoy!

Per Serving: Calories: 144
Protein: 5g
Carbohydrates: 29g
Fat: 1g
Cholesterol: 0mg
Sodium: 265mg
Potassium: 388mg
Phosphorus: 92mg
Calcium: 169mg
Fiber: 4g

Soft Red Cabbage with Cranberry

SERVES 5 / PREP TIME: 15 MINUTES / COOK TIME: 1 HOUR

A mix of sweet and tart flavors. Try this as a side dish for Thanksgiving.

---

2 red cabbages
1 cup of canned cranberries, juices
drained
1 tsp. of balsamic vinegar
1 tsp. of allspice
1 tsp. of ground black pepper
1 tsp. of brown sugar substitute
2 cups of water

---

1. Wash and slice the red cabbage, making sure it's not too thin.
2. Throw all of the ingredients into the slow cooker.
3. Cook on Low for 1 hour or until the cabbage is soft.
4. Enjoy this as a main dish with rice or noodles or as a side dish.

Per Serving: Calories: 107
Protein: 2g
Carbohydrates: 27g
Fat: 0g
Cholesterol: 0mg
Sodium: 50mg
Potassium: 335mg
Phosphorus: 44mg
Calcium: 67mg
Fiber: 4g

Slow Cooked Cabbage with Cucumber and Dill Relish

SERVES 4 / PREP TIME: 5 MINUTES / COOK TIME: 1.5 HOURS

The tender slow cooked cabbage is complemented with a cool, crisp relish for something a little different.

1 white cabbage
1 tbsp. of olive oil
1 lemon, juice squeezed
A pinch of black pepper
1 cucumber, diced
1 tbsp. of fresh or dried dill

1. Slice the cabbage into strips.
2. Melt the butter in a skillet over a medium heat and add the juice from half of the lemon (save one half for serving).
3. Pour this into the slow cooker and add in the cabbage.
4. Cover with a little water, just to reach the top of the cabbage.
5. Cook on a Low with the lid on for 1 ½ hours.
6. Remove the lid and continue to cook if it's still a bit watery for 10 minutes.
7. Prepare your salad by dicing the cucumber and mixing in the dill.
8. Squeeze the leftover lemon juice into the salad.
9. Serve a helping of the cabbage with the cool cucumber relish.

Per Serving: Calories: 73
Protein: 2g
Carbohydrates: 10g
Fat: 4g
Cholesterol: 0mg
Sodium: 13mg
Potassium: 375mg
Phosphorus: 61mg
Calcium: 80mg
Fiber: 3g

SOUPS, STOCKS & SIDES

Tarragon, Carrot & Lemon Soup

SERVES 4 / PREP TIME: 15 MINUTES / COOK TIME: 7-8 HOURS

A lovely hot, warming soup with a little added zest.

1 tbsp. of olive oil
1 tsp. of mustard seeds, ground
1 tsp. of fennel seeds, ground
1 tbsp. of oregano
1 tbsp. of ground ginger
6 medium carrots, peeled and chopped
1 red onion, diced
1 lemon, zest and juice

4 cups of water
1 tsp. of ground black pepper

1. Heat the oil in a skillet over a medium heat.
2. Once hot, add the mustard and fennel seeds.
3. Cook them for just a minute.
4. Add the ginger and cook for another minute.
5. Add the carrots, onions and lemon juice.
6. Cook them for at least 5 minutes or until the vegetables are soft.
7. Add all the cooked ingredients to the slow cooker.
8. Add in the water and the oregano, too.
9. Cook on Low for about 7-8 hours.
10. Serve with the black pepper sprinkled on top.

Per Serving : Calories: 99
Protein: 2g
Carbohydrates: 26g
Fat: 4g
Cholesterol: 0mg
Sodium: 68mg
Potassium: 378mg
Phosphorus: 58mg
Calcium: 87mg
Fiber: 5g

Thai-Infused Turkey Soup

SERVES 6 /   PREP TIME: 15 MINUTES /   COOK TIME: 4-6 HOURS

Full of bold, zesty flavors to add a twist to a wholesome turkey soup.

½ stick of lemongrass, sliced
1 tbsp. of cilantro
1 red chili, finely chopped
1 tbsp. of coconut oil
1 tbsp. of oregano
1 white onion, chopped
1 garlic clove, minced
1 tbsp. of ground ginger

12oz of skinless turkey breast, diced
½ cup of water
½ cup of low-sodium chicken stock
1 fresh lime, juiced
½ cup of pak choy leaves, shredded
1 cup of canned water chestnuts
2 green onions, chopped

1. Crush the lemongrass, cilantro, chili, coconut oil and oregano in a blender or pestle and mortar to form a paste.
2. Heat a large pan/wok with 1 tbsp. coconut oil on a high heat.
3. Sauté the onions, garlic and ginger until soft.
4. Add the turkey cubes and brown evenly on each side.
5. Add the water and stir. Now add the paste.
6. Slowly add the stock until a broth is formed.
7. Now add all of the ingredients from the wok to the slow cooker.
8. Squeeze in the lime juice.
9. Cook everything on Low for 4-6 hours.
10. Add the pak choy and water chestnuts 20 minutes before serving.
11. Serve steaming with the green onion sprinkled over the top.

Per Serving: Calories: 115
Protein: 13g
Carbohydrates: 10g
Fat: 3g
Cholesterol: 32mg
Sodium: 37mg
Potassium: 323mg
Phosphorus: 122mg
Calcium: 47mg
Fiber: 2g

Tender Pork & White Cabbage Soup

SERVES 6 / PREP TIME: 10 MINUTES / COOK TIME: 7-8 HOURS

A classic mix of soft, succulent pork and cabbage for a warming, hearty soup.

½ tbsp. of olive oil
½ red onion, chopped
1 garlic cloves, minced
6oz of lean pork loin
½ cup of low-sodium chicken stock
1 cup of water
½ tbsp. of allspice
½ cup of white cabbage, sliced
½ tsp. of black pepper

1. Trim the fat from the pork loin meat and slice into 1 inch thick slices.
2. Heat up the oil in a wok.
3. Add the onion and garlic and sauté for 5 minutes on a low heat.
4. Add the pork to the wok and cook for 7-8 minutes to brown.
5. Transfer the ingredients from the wok to the slow cooker.
6. Pour the stock and water into the slow cooker.
7. Add in the allspice to season.
8. Add the in sliced cabbage and stir the pot well.
9. Cook on Low for a further 7-8 hours until the pork is very soft.
10. Sprinkle with the black pepper to finish.

Per Serving: Calories: 84
Protein: 14g
Carbohydrates: 3g
Fat: 4g
Cholesterol: 22.5mg
Sodium: 117mg
Potassium: 187.5mg
Phosphorus: 85.5mg
Calcium: 21.5mg
Fiber: 0.5g

Slow Cooked Vegetable Stock

SERVES 10 / PREP TIME: 10 MINUTES / COOK TIME: 4-6 HOURS

A stock recipe that can be prepared overnight!

---

2 onions, diced
3 carrots, peeled and chopped
3 celery stalks, chopped
1 garlic clove
1 bay leaf
1 tbsp. of rosemary
1 tbsp. of oregano

1 tbsp. of dried parsley
1 tsp. of whole black peppercorns
5 cups of water
1 tbsp. of olive oil

---

1. Peel and roughly chop the vegetables.
2. Soak them in warm water for 10 minutes.
3. Add the vegetables, garlic, herbs and peppercorns into the slow cooker.
4. Fill up the slow cooker with boiling water and add the oil.
5. Cook on High for roughly 4-6 hours.
6. Strain the stock using a sieve.
7. Use immediately or allow to it cool and refrigerate.
8. If refrigerated, use within 2-3 days or freeze for 3-4 weeks in a sealed container.

Per Serving: Calories: 41
Protein: 1g
Carbohydrates: 7g
Fat: 2g
Cholesterol: 0mg
Sodium: 22mg
Potassium: 153mg
Phosphorus: 24mg
Calcium: 29mg
Fiber: 2g

Slow Cooked Chicken Stock

SERVES 30 / PREP TIME: 5 MINUTES / COOK TIME: 40 MINUTES

It's so simple to cook this stock up in your slow cooker!

1/2 stick lemon-grass, finely sliced
1 tbsp cilantro
1 green chili, finely chopped
1 tbsp coconut oil
1/4 cup fresh basil leaves
1 white onion, chopped
1 garlic clove, minced
1 thumb size piece of minced ginger
4oz skinless turkey breasts, sliced
4 cups water
1 cup canned water chestnuts, drained
2 scallions, chopped
1 fresh lime

1. Crush the lemon-grass, cilantro, chili, 1 tbsp oil and basil leaves in a blender or pestle and mortar to form a paste.
2. Heat a large pan/wok with 1 tbsp olive oil on a high heat.
3. Sauté the onions, garlic and ginger until soft.
4. Add the turkey and brown each side for 4-5 minutes.
5. Add the broth and stir.
6. Now add the paste and stir.
7. Next add the water chestnuts, turn down the heat slightly and allow to simmer for 25-30 minutes or until turkey is thoroughly cooked through.
8. Serve hot with the green onion sprinkled over the top.

Per Serving: Calories 123
Protein 10 g
Carbohydrates 12 g
Fat 3 g
Sodium 501 mg
Potassium 151 mg
Phosphorus 110 mg

Lime Rice with Coconut & Chili

SERVES 5 / PREP TIME: 15 MINUTES / COOK TIME: 2 HOURS

Mild, tangy and with a little bit of zest. This is a perfect base to add a little extra flavor to your favorite rice dishes.

2 tbsp. of olive oil
2 green onions, thinly sliced
1 red chilli, seeded and finely diced
1 clove of garlic, minced
2 tbsp. of unsalted butter
2 cups of white rice
1 lime, juiced
½ stick of lemon grass, finely chopped

2 bay leaves
1 cup of coconut milk (unenriched)
2 cups of water
1 tsp. of ground black pepper

1. Preheat the slow cooker to Low.
2. Heat the oil in a wok over a high heat and add the onions, chilli and garlic.
3. Cook and for 5 minutes until the onions soften but aren't brown.
4. Add the butter and stir in the rice for 2-3 minutes to warm it through.
5. Turn the heat up to high.
6. Add in the lime, lemongrass, bay leaves, coconut milk and water.
7. Transfer everything to the slow cooker.
8. Cover it up and cook for 2 hours, stirring after the first hour.
9. Sprinkle with the ground black pepper to serve.

Per Serving: Calories: 247
Protein: 3g
Carbohydrates: 22g
Fat: 17g
Cholesterol: 0mg
Sodium: 11mg
Potassium: 194mg
Phosphorus: 82mg
Calcium: 33mg
Fiber: 2g

Slow Roasted Beets with Lemon and Honey

SERVES 5 / PREP TIME: 5 MINUTES / COOK TIME: 6-7 HOURS

Roasting the beets brings out the sweet, mellow flavour, perfect for a side or added to other dishes.

2 tbsp. of olive oil
10 medium beets (approx. 4 pounds),
trimmed and peeled
1/3 cup of water
2 tbsp. of honey
2 tbsp. of cider vinegar
½ tsp. of garlic powder
1 lemon, juiced
A pinch of freshly ground pepper

1. Rub the inside of your slow cooker with olive oil.
2. Add the beets to the bottom of the slow cooker.
3. In a small bowl, whisk together the remaining ingredients and pour over the beets.
4. Cover and cook on Low for 6-7 hours until the beets are very soft.
5. Remove the beets from the slow cooker and slice them.
6. (Hint: You could blend these in a food processor to make a delicious puree to add to meats, fish or vegetables.)

Per Serving: Calories: 129
Protein: 2g
Carbohydrates: 20g
Fat: 6g
Cholesterol: 0mg
Sodium: 94mg
Potassium: 382mg
Phosphorus: 48mg
Calcium: 23mg
Fiber: 2g

Slow Cooked Sweet Onion Relish

SERVES 4 / PREP TIME: 10 MINUTES / COOK TIME: 40 MINUTES

Amazing!

---

1 tbsp olive oil
3 onions, peeled and thinly sliced
1 tsp brown sugar
2 garlic cloves, minced
1 tbsp plain flour
1 cup low-sodium beef stock, hot
2 cups water
1 slice of white bread, cubed into croutons

---

1. Add the oil in a saucepan (with a lid) over a medium heat.
2. Sweat the onions for 2 minutes before adding the lid and leaving for 5-7 minutes until tender.
3. Remove the lid and sprinkle over the sugar.
4. Stir continuously for a few minutes until onions are golden brown and caramelized.
5. Now add the garlic and flour and stir.
6. Turn up the heat slightly.
7. Slowly add the beef stock and water whilst stirring.
8. Cover and simmer for 20 minutes.
9. Meanwhile, toast or grill the ciabatta croutons.
10. Serve the soup with a sprinkle of croutons and enjoy!

Per Serving: Calories 152
Protein 1 g
Carbohydrates 3 g
Fat 7 g
Sodium 5 mg
Potassium 59 mg
Phosphorus 29 mg

Poached Spiced Apples & Pears

SERVES 4 / PREP TIME: 5 MINUTES / COOK TIME: 7-8 HOURS

Sweet and fragrantly spiced for a delicious dessert.

2 apples, peeled and halved
2 pears, peeled and halved
1 tbsp. of cloves
1 tsp. of allspice

1 cinnamon stick
1 tsp. of brown sugar

1. Turn the slow cooker to a low setting.
2. Peel and half the apples and pears.
3. Poke the cloves into the flesh of the fruits at even spaces.
4. Place into the slow cooker and cover with water.
5. Add the allspice, cinnamon stick and the brown sugar. Mix.
6. Cover and cook for about 7-8 hours.
7. Serve however you like.
8. (Hint: It works especially well with crumbled ginger cookies on the top.)

Per Serving: Calories: 73
Protein: 0g
Carbohydrates: 19g
Fat: 0g
Cholesterol: 0mg
Sodium: 3mg
Potassium: 138mg
Phosphorus: 17mg
Calcium: 19mg
Fiber: 4g

Honey & Mustard Glazed Root Vegetables

SERVES 5 / PREP TIME: 5 MINUTES / COOK TIME: 7-8 HOURS

Slow roasted root vegetables with a tangy sweet glaze.

---

4 medium carrots, peeled and roughly chopped
2 cups of rutabaga, peeled and chunked
1 tbsp. of mustard
2 tbsp. of honey
½ cup. of water
1 tbsp. of unsalted butter

A pinch of ground black pepper

---

1. Place all of the ingredients in the slow cooker and stir well.
2. Cover and cook on Low for 7 to 8 hours.
3. When the vegetables are tender, serve as a side or with fluffy rice.

Per Serving: Calories: 89
Protein: 1g
Carbohydrates: 17g
Fat: 3g
Cholesterol: 6mg
Sodium: 63mg
Potassium: 333mg
Phosphorus: 55mg
Calcium: 51mg
Fiber: 3g

CONVERSION TABLES

Volume

Imperial	Metric
1 tbsp	15ml
2 fl oz	55 ml
3 fl oz	75 ml
5 fl oz (¼ pint)	150 ml
10 fl oz (½ pint)	275 ml
1 pint	570 ml
1 ¼ pints	725 ml
1 ¾ pints	1 litre
2 pints	1.2 litres
2½ pints	1.5 litres
4 pints	2.25 litres

Oven temperatures

Gas Mark	Fahrenheit	Celsius
1/4	225	110
1/2	250	130
1	275	140
2	300	150
3	325	170
4	350	180
5	375	190
6	400	200
7	425	220
8	450	230
9	475	240

Weight

Imperial	Metric
½ oz	10 g
¾ oz	20 g
1 oz	25 g
1½ oz	40 g
2 oz	50 g
2½ oz	60 g
3 oz	75 g
4 oz	110 g
4½ oz	125 g
5 oz	150 g
6 oz	175 g
7 oz	200 g
8 oz	225 g
9 oz	250 g
10 oz	275 g
12 oz	350 g

BIBLIOGRAPHY

Schoenfeld, Brad, Alan Aragon, and James W. Krieger. "The Effect of Protein Timing on Muscle Strength and Hypertrophy: A Meta-analysis." J Int Soc Sports Nutr Journal of the International Society of Sports Nutrition 10, no. 1 (2013): 53. doi:10.1186/1550-2783-10-53.

Jacobs, Peter, and Lucille Wood. Macro-nutrients. St. Louis, MO: Mosby, 2004.

Kumar, V., P. Atherton, K. Smith, and M. J. Rennie. "Human Muscle Protein Synthesis and Breakdown during and after Exercise." Journal of Applied Physiology 106, no. 6 (2009): 2026-039. doi:10.1152/japplphysiol.91481.2008.

Langley-Evans, Simon. "Keith N. Frayn Metabolic Regulation: A Human Perspective, 2nd Ed. Oxford, UK: Blackwell Publishing 2003. P. 339. £24.99 (paperback). ISBN 0-632-06384-X." BJN British Journal of Nutrition 92, no. 06 (2004): 1013. doi:10.1079/bjn20041232.

Rickli, Jonas. "Bodybuilding." Grenzbereiche Der Sportmedizin, 1990, 159-76. doi:10.1007/978-3-642-75429-6_11.

"Understanding Bodybuilding." Science Signaling 2004, no. 239 (2004). doi:10.1126/stke.2392004tw227.

Lacovara, Paul Dominick. Bodybuilding. 2002.

Gilman, Sander L. Diets and Dieting: A Cultural Encyclopedia. New York: Routledge, 2008.

INDEX

45352935R00127

Made in the USA
Middletown, DE
01 July 2017